Tai Chi

Tai Chi

DANNY CONNOR

with Marnix Wells and Michael Tse

STANLEY PAUL

LONDON · SYDNEY · AUCKLAND · JOHANNESBURG

Stanley Paul & Co. Ltd
An imprint of Random House
20 Vauxhall Bridge Road, London SW1V 2SA

Random House Australia (Pty) Ltd
20 Alfred Street, Milsons Point, Sydney 2061

Random House New Zealand Limited
PO Box 40-086, Glenfield, Auckland 10

Random House South Africa (Pty) Ltd
PO Box 337, Bergvlei 2012, South Africa

First published 1989
Reprinted 1991, 1993 (twice), 1995

© Danny Connor 1989

Set in Optima by Tek Art Ltd

Printed and bound in Great Britain by
Scotprint Ltd, Musselburgh, Scotland

British Library Cataloguing in Publication Data
Connor, Danny
  Tai chi.
  1. T'ai Chi ch'uan – manuals
  I. Title
  796.8'155
  ISBN 0 09 173983 7

Contents

Acknowledgements

Marnix Wells for his enormous input with regard to the translations and interpretations from the original Chinese text, and for the benefit of his vast experience in a field where few Chinese scholars dare to tread.

Michael Tse for his patience and skill in coaching me in the *Taiji Qigong* section, and for his remarkable ability which has touched many people's lives.

Mr Mun from the Beijing Physical Culture Institute who taught me the 24-step tai-chi.

Loh Tsu Hun who taught me the 37-step tai-chi in Singapore and encouraged me on my journey.

My sister, Pat Cronshaw, who 'minded the shop' for many years, whilst I travelled Asia acquiring knowledge in this field.

Moira Shawcross, Patricia Bryan and Christine Kirk for their fine editing and excellent typing skills.

Joanna Connor who took time out from minding our two sons Alexander and Lucas to help with the two person exercise.

Brian Seabright who held off the phone calls whilst I was writing this book.

Trevor Griffiths and Gill Cliff for their encouragement over the years.

Alan Seabright for his fine photography.

Roddy Bloomfield and Dominique Shead for convincing me that I should do it.

Marion Paull for her editor's advice and Louise Speller for her final edit and patience.

All the unsung people who help to make up a book and sell it.

Last but not least, the Teddy boy I bumped into on a Number 19 bus in Manchester 30 years ago, who set me on strange journey of discovery.

Foreword

Five years ago, I invited the author of this book to join me in America to help me prepare and stage a Tai-chi sequence to end my play *Real Dreams*. The idea for such an ending, the metaphor it sought to actualise, emerged from the hundreds of hours of usually through-the-night discourses that Danny and I have had over many years; so it seemed fitting he should be the one to flesh it out.

In fewer than thirty days, at usually not more than an hour a day with the cast, he not only taught twelve very singular young American actors a form of 24-step tai-chi but also created a closing scene of startling grace and rivetting intensity. Trying to sum up the experience some months later, one of the young actors wrote: 'The pupil's only gift to the great teacher is to learn. Danny's passion for the art and his belief in the practice made *not* making that gift unthinkable.'

Those same qualities of passion and belief, framed here on the page by Danny's inimitable clarity and humour, inform the book he has written and make it a considerable pleasure to read.

Let learning commence.

Trevor Griffiths

BOSTON SPA 27 AUGUST 1989

Introduction

Tai-chi is philosophy in movement, a combination of ancient exercises intertwined with Taoist philosophy, also practised as a martial art of high technique. I hope to cover in this book some of the history, theory, basic practice, health, philosophy, meditation as well as my own personal experiences.

Tai-chi being a gateway to the inner self, it ideally reflects our time. The Chinese have known for centuries the benefit of such therapeutic gymnastics, and their growing popularity reflects the current criticism of impact aerobics.

The 'hard' and 'soft' styles of Chinese martial arts have ebbed and flowed in popularity over the centuries. There is a pulse nowadays towards the 'yin' element – female/nurturing – as opposed to the 'yang' element – male/aggressive. The world is becoming green in its consciousness, and this concept of preservation is becoming internalized through the practice of tai-chi and qigong. Many thousands have benefited through meditation here in the UK. Tai-chi may be termed moving meditation and gives a balance to static practice.

I would like to apologise to all my teachers for the audacity in presenting a book whilst they live. The publishers resisted my entreaties to use drawings instead of photographs, and looking at my photographs I can only see where my technique falls short of that which I have witnessed. I can only hope that it may awaken people's interest in what I have found an interesting subject for over twenty years. In my studies I have always been fascinated by skills that may be retained into dotage; for me it's like having a companion that emerges at my will. At the least, as was once said of opium, 'it kills the ennui'. Tai-chi allows you to enter into your own company and experientially know yourself.

Tai-chi is one of the five Chinese accomplishments, the other four being painting, poetry, calligraphy, and music. These are reputed to be the qualities of the 'superior man'. (Interestingly in Chinese 'he' and 'she' pronouns are pronounced the same.)

Back to the book, I have shown some two person exercises (thanks Joanna!). If you can find a compliant partner they add an interesting dimension to the practice.

The chapters on Great Polarity boxing and the Thirteen Actions will be of interest to all existing tai-chi students for whom they are not commonly available in print and offer to them further contemplation of their chosen art. The tai-chi qigong section I offer for immediate practice so that the benefits may be enjoyed by all.

I have compiled a list of interesting books on the subject that I have read. There are many other good books on tai-chi available which I have not included which cover the various systems and methods of tai-chi. I in no way wish to denigrate the quality of those books by their omission.

If in some way this book stimulates your interest and guides you to a good teacher then it will have served its purpose.

I have produced a video tape which includes the 24-step tai-chi and the 18-movement tai-chi qigong. This is available from: Oriental World, 18 Swan Street, Manchester M4 5JN, price £19.95 incl. postage for those wishing to study in more detail.

1   What is Tai-chi

Tai-chi, as practised in China and now increasingly popular in the West, is a unique system of exercise based on the principles of relaxed breathing, rhythmical movement and balance. It also serves as a method of self-defence.

According to legend, this 'internal' or Taoist boxing was first developed during the Sung dynasty (AD 960–1279) by the alchemist Chang-San-feng, lived on Wu-dang Mountain in Hupei Province.

Modern historians, however, trace tai-chi's origins to the Chen village in Henan Province during the late Ming and early Qing dynasties, some 350 years ago.

Invasions and domestic uprisings disseminated many forms of boxing and martial arts throughout China. Whilst previous methods emphasized vigorous blows and quick movements, this new style incorporated the principle of subduing the 'hard' within the 'soft', as well as the martial saying about defeating the force of 1000 pounds with the action of 4 ounces.

Tai-chi's fusion of energetic and relaxed movements, flowing together seamlessly, is often referred to as *chang chuan* 'long boxing', and likened to the endless winding and flowing of the Yangtze river.

It is generally accepted that this new method was an adaptation of selected aspects of boxing styles that were popular during the Ming dynasty. The new principles, such as 'adapting to the style of others' and 'sticking' to the opponent became popular among the people and were contrary to the hard Shaolin methods which prevailed at the time.

In the late eighteenth century, a tai-chi master by the name of Wang Zongyue summed up this new boxing style by relating the principles to the central theory of Taoism (Daoism), which incorporates the principles of Yin and Yang (the two opposing and interdependent principles in nature: the former feminine and passive, the latter masculine and active). This method of boxing became known as *tai-chi chuan*.

Up to this point, tai-chi had been practised mainly in the province of Henan, but in the middle of the nineteenth century, a tai-chi master by the name of Yang Lu-chan brought tai-chi to Peking and soon it began to spread throughout China.

Since then, tai-chi has undergone many changes. Different styles have emerged. Movements have tended to become more relaxed and graceful, many of the foot-stamping, leaps and explosive techniques have disappeared and, apparently as a result, its popularity with young and old alike has increased. The health benefits of tai-chi are now widely appreciated. There has been much research surrounding its therapeutic benefits and this is referred to in a later chapter.

2 A First Encounter

My first exposure to tai-chi occurred, strangely enough, in Japan during a period in my life when I was studying karate. The year was 1967 and I had been accepted at Nihon University to study the wado-ryu style. I found the training arduous and my health began to suffer; my weight dropped from 160 lbs to 130 lbs.

To supplement my income I began to teach English conversation, meeting up with other expatriates who plied their accents in a similar manner. I joined them for dinner and opposite the café in which we ate was a building where, whilst wrestling with chopsticks, I observed a group on the first floor practising tai-chi.

This was my first sighting of tai-chi's slow, mesmerizing movements. My first thought was 'How can it possibly be a martial art, when everyone is moving in slow motion?'

My friend Jimmy Mathie, who was a student of kendo at the time remarked, 'Perhaps they move slowly to get more out of it, just as chewing your food slowly gives you more benefit!' I couldn't argue the logic of this, but I still had trouble equating this to a martial context. I had to admit that the movements had a roundness and balance that I found absorbing, and the mood displayed by those practising seemed calm and possessed and more akin to a tea ceremony than to martial application.

Until this point, all my studies had centred around karate, which lays such great emphasis on speed and power. For weeks I watched the group performing with increasing interest and irritation; unknown to my conscious mind, I was being seduced by the calmness and balance I was witnessing. Daily I became more and more entranced by the subtlety of the exercise and against a part of myself I went upstairs and watched the group practise their 'weird' exercise.

The teacher was a middle-aged Chinese named Zhang Yizhong, a student of the renowned master Wang Shujin from mainland China. I was to meet Wang-Shu-Jing later, through his student Marnix St John Wells (a friend and collaborator in much of this book), who is himself a Chinese scholar and author of *The Dragon's Hum*.

It would appear that the main reason I began studying tai-chi parallels that of many other people . . . health! I still wished to develop my martial skills and slowly I began to discover that *tai-chi chuan* ('grand ultimate boxing') was a martial art *par excellence*. I blessed my luck that fortune had blown me along a path which opened the door to this treasure house of Chinese culture.

My first thought was to learn the skills and translate them through my knowledge of karate, but the technqiues have a rounded quality which karate does not share, so I quickly had to abandon that approach.

I found that I had difficulty in keeping my hands open, due to excessive punching practice in karate training. So much of my psyche was connected to the security of my fist, which had until then served my ego so well. Tai-chi presented a problem that I had not anticipated!

The reality was that I had reached a crossroads in my martial studies – a choice had to be made. In retrospect, I realize I had already made the decision. Probably it was the fact that Zhang Yizhong had invited all visitors to the gymnasium to punch him in the stomach and none had managed to have any effect on his composure. This demonstration impressed me greatly and gave encouragement to my studies. This group must have been amongst the first to practise in Japan, and I studied with them for some time.

My fellow student and friend Bruce 'Kumar' Frantzis, now a noted 'wu' style tai-chi instructor, had already made the transition from karate to tai-chi. In his search for quality instruction Bruce brought over from Taipei a young Taiwanese named Liao Wei Shan, who had extraordinary skills at 'pushing hands' (tai-chi sparring). His skill was such that during practice he sent us flying against the walls through his ability to uproot our balance.

Bruce would deliver full-blooded knee kicks to show what his new find could withstand. On one occasion, he struck so hard that Liao's spectacles flew off and landed on the other side of the room. Liao was nonplussed and walked across the room to retrieve them, sat down and carried on talking. Both Bruce and I were mightily impressed by this exhibition of 'inner strength'. It was years later that I found out that this ability to absorb blows is part of the qigong 'breathing skill' method. This particular ability is known as 'iron-shirt qigong' and is a separate practice to tai-chi itself.

In 1969 I found myself in Singapore, the 'Lion City', and decided to continue my tai-chi studies there. At the time, Asia was in the grip of Bruce Lee fever and the martial arts were becoming very popular. *Tae kwon do* (Korean karate) attracted the most interest, probably because of its penchant for high kicking, by means of which practitioners sought to emulate the new hero Bruce Lee (otherwise known as the Little Dragon).

I joined a so called tai-chi club that had caught the fever and the first night saw me, along with the rest of the class, jumping against a plank leaning against a wall. I decided this wasn't what I was looking for, and so visited a number of other groups that didn't seem to suit me either and began to feel depressed at not finding a suitable teacher. Then someone told me of a teacher named Loh Tsu Hun. I went along with an optimistic air and knocked on his door.

A pleasant-faced, healthy-looking man in his late twenties answered my knock. 'I'd like to learn tai-chi,' I said, as I gave him my letter of introduction.

'I don't teach anymore, I'm too busy,' he replied.

I was disappointed, but he was polite and apologized that his work as a schoolteacher had caused him to stop his other teaching, and so I left. One thing about learning Chinese skills is that you can't force anyone to teach you if they don't want to. There is a Chinese saying, 'It's hard to find a good teacher, it's even harder to find a good student.'

I have since found out that the traditional method of approaching a teacher is to take a present to introduce yourself. Historically, this used to be tea . . . and the price of some Chinese teas can take your breath away. The modern approach is to make a cash gift inside a red envelope. This process is best conducted after an introduction by a third party who recommends you. There is no equivalent, in Western culture, to this attempt to win acceptance by a teacher who holds the key to the skills you desire. Generally the payment is not fixed, but is according to the means of the student. If you are looking for quality though, the last thing you need is for the teacher to think you're a cheapskate!

I left Mr Loh and trudged home through the alleys, but something told me that he wasn't being exactly frank in his explanation. He looked too calm and non-committal and I could tell by his bearing that he was still practising. He had the demeanour of someone balanced and at ease with himself.

I related what had happened at the meeting to the friend who had given me Loh Tsu Hun's name and I asked where he taught. I was taken along to a new address and found myself in a courtyard, dominated by a giant banyan tree which had surely been there at least 100 years before the British Empire reached Singapore.

Although no one was there, I felt comfortable and decided to wait. It was a haven of peace after the bustle of the Singapore traffic and embodied the atmosphere that I felt would be conducive to practising tai-chi.

Two youths in their early teens came into the courtyard and looked at me strangely. They unlocked the door of a small building in the corner of the yard, then emerged carrying sweeping brushes and still giving me odd glances. They must have held a small meeting in the hut, for they came over to where I was sitting. Mustering their linguistic skills they said, 'Yes? Yes, can we help?'

'I'm waiting for Mr Loh Tsu Hun,' I replied.

'What for?' they asked.

I was a foreigner, and they were clearly suspicious.

'I wish to learn tai-chi.'

'Oh!' they said, evidently relieved to have found the purpose of my visit. The threat of my presence seemed to diminish.

Just then, Mr Loh turned the corner into the yard and spied me talking to the two juniors, who jumped up and ran over to tell him who, what, etc. He waved them away and came over with a half smile on his face.

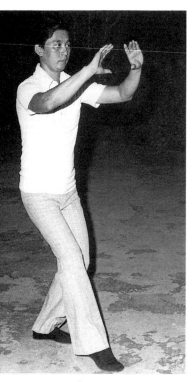

Loh Tsu Hun, my tai-chi teacher in Singapore, seen here performing a movement from liu-her-pa-fa (six directions eight harmonies' style of internal boxing)

'So you came, eh?' he said. He looked at me for a while, scratched his head. 'OK, I suppose. How long are you going to stay in Singapore and when can you begin to study?'

'I'm staying for a year and I can study whenever you say.'

'Monday, Wednesday, Friday, 7 p.m.'

'Thank you,' I said. He told me the monthly fee to the Athletic Association, which I now forget, and we shook hands. I thanked him again and left with my spirits raised, congratulating myself on my good fortune at securing a teacher with the bearing of a traditional Chinese gentleman.

I studied with Loh Tsu Hun both privately and with the group for a year and practised daily at 7 a.m. He taught me the 37–step Yang style which had been devised by Cheng Man-ching. I practised regularly and he seemed pleased with my progress.

Sometimes, if it rained, he would take me to a local tea shop and I would ask him many questions about the Chinese arts. He was generous with his explanations. Mr Loh had been educated at a Chinese school, but English was his second language and he had a good command of it. I learned from him much about the history of the Chinese martial arts and the principles behind them.

He told me that the best time to practise was between 6 and 8 a.m. because extra vitamin D may be absorbed during these early-morning hours. The Chinese have been practising in this way for hundreds of years, long before modern science discovered vitamins.

During this period I was living in a rambling, old-style, high-ceilinged house with a Chinese family who temporarily adopted me. The family consisted of a typical three generations with an assortment of uncles, one of whom practised tai-chi every morning. I could never bring myself to practise with him, however, because of the unusual rhythm with which he performed his round of tai-chi. His method appeared 'external' in quality, and I later discovered that he was a former quickstep-dancing champion of Singapore! (I later found out that Bruce Lee was the cha-cha champion of Hong Kong – maybe some connection there!).

Chinese martial arts are commonly divided into two different schools, the external being the shaolin method where the student practises vigorous forms displaying speed, strength and courage. The three internal schools, tai-chi, bagua and hsing-i, are practised in a more relaxed manner and each have the mind as the central point.

Tai-chi has as its symbol the Yin Yang which connects it with the study of Taoism. Bagua, involves walking in a circle with smooth interconnecting steps and hand movement, depicted symbolically with the hexagrams which connect it with the I-ching (the book of changes). Hsing-i has a basic five-fist method, which is related to the five elements, wood, earth, metal, fire and water, which in turn relate to Chinese medical and philosophical theory.

Nowadays in New China wu-shu students learn both the acrobatic external forms and also the 'internal' for display. Many purists feel that this act of 'performing' the 'internal' loses the 'I' or mind behind the action and consider the performing of them to be the same as putting them in aspic, although aspic does act as a preserver.

Youth by its nature and energy is competitive and we as students were no different as we disputed daily the differences in our learned techniques, rather than the similarities.

This was for a time a frustrating period, as it challenged what I was learning. Many people who study tai-chi are disappointed to discover that there are different styles, while feeling that theirs is the 'true path'. I imagine the same problem exists for those who convert to Christianity, Islam or Buddhism only to find out that they all enjoy the vagaries and interpretations of different individuals.

One day I felt I had made a huge jump in my comprehension of tai-chi principles. Up to this point I was immovable in my arguments and realized that I was still 'external' in my approach and that I was still applying my karate psychology, rather than the taoist precepts of 'non-action' and non-resistance to achieve success.

The term 'letting go' is considered by many in the West to be an act of sacrifice, but the letting go of old precepts that are holding you back is one of the most liberating of experiences. To this day, seventeen years later, I remember the room, the lighting and where I was standing. Everything is still so vivid, as realization dawned and a state of ecstasy engulfed me. I believe I experienced the state known in Zen meditation as 'Satori' or enlightenment, and it all came about because one day my Chinese cousin Victor looked at me in the middle of one of our tai-chi arguments and said, 'We're not in competition, you know!'

I was struck dumb by his comment and a most unusual feeling of excitement came over me. I suddenly had to be alone and went into the courtyard at the back of the house, where I could see the sky; the most exquisite feeling flooded through my body, leaving me tingling all over. I looked around and everything seemed so perfect. I felt I was dissolving; tears welled up and the words, 'not in competition' echoed in my brain. I felt completely relaxed and taking a breath, I shuddered with excitement. I felt my body drinking air, cool and fresh and sweet. I believe for a moment I was without any sense of self, in harmony with the universe, in a state of ecstasy that had no duality, no conflict.

The whole experience lasted only about fifteen seconds. I tried to hold on to the feeling, but slowly I returned to the 'real' world. For a moment there, I believe I experienced something transcendental. I think that at that moment I felt what other people have described more poetically, that sense of 'letting go'. It was, for me, a release of an inner conflict with the principles of tai-chi. After that I was able to practise with a lighter heart.

Even now that experience remains clear in my mind. No past, no future, just the present . . . triggered by a simple comment. For the first time in my life I felt alive in the deepest sense of the word.

I returned to the U K in 1972, after five years' absence, in time to witness the kung fu boom. Both Bruce Lee and the TV series *Kung Fu*, starring David Carradine as Kwai Chan Kane, had invaded the psyche of British youth and virtually overnight two new words had entered the language.

I began to hold tai-chi classes in Manchester, but I longed to continue my studies. I heard of a Chinese lady who taught at

Durham University. Her name was Rose Li and she was a scholar of Chinese who had had the good fortune to study with a tai-chi master in Peking before the Revolution. She was recognized for her ability in the three internal systems: xing-yi (mind boxing), bagua and tai-chi. Even though middle-aged, she could still place her toe on her forehead.

I persuaded her to come to Manchester to hold weekly classes. Her teachings gave me much information with regard to the 'internal' martial arts and Chinese etiquette. Her gentle coaxing and subtle method influenced me greatly and I learned many things that could so easily have been missed. It was a joy to study with her for over a year.

Eventually her talents were called for in London and to the best of my knowledge, she still teaches a small coterie of students in the London area.

In 1957 Mao Tse Tung gave his famous order to 'let a hundred blossoms bloom'; and *wu-shu*, the Chinese martial arts, had taken off in a big way. Wu-shu was adopted as a national sport, which preserved the martial arts within a gymnastic aspect.

In 1972, Nixon's visit to China opened the 'bamboo curtain' and after a visit by a Chinese wu-shu troupe to the U K, I was able to obtain an address in China to which I could apply to further my studies.

I wrote to the Peking Physical Culture Institute and was invited to attend. I flew from Hong Kong to Peking, excited to be visiting the Middle Kingdom for the first time.

I caught a taxi from the airport and arrived at the Institute during siesta which was from 12 until 3 p.m. China at this time was beginning to emerge from its isolation and I was the first British person to study at the Institute. Nowadays regular courses for foreigners are held during holiday periods. Located twelve miles from the centre of Peking it is surrounded by fields where life had not changed for decades. I felt I was truly in China with buffalo carts and bicycles everywhere. Those were the days of the 'iron ricebowl', when everyone had a job for life. Officials at the Institute went into a flat spin at the arrival of this foreigner two days before he was due. They managed to find an English speaker who remonstrated with me for arriving too early! At this time, barely a handful of foreigners had attended their wu-shu courses.

They quickly arranged a group of teachers to interview me; I was informed that I would have to show them the tai-chi that I knew.

I was nervous in front of all the institute instructors. After they had watched my performance, I was relieved to hear (through the interpreter), that my tai-chi could be 'repaired'. I was told that I would study with Mr Mun, who had assisted in the formation of the 48-step tai-chi and was one of the Institute's senior instructors. It was decided that my study would begin at 8 a.m. and would resume in the afternoon after siesta.

My first few days were spent learning to walk in the tai-chi manner – which left my legs seriously aching, and made walking downstairs from the dormitory to the refectory enormously difficult. After the first day's four-hour practice, I had to hold on to the bannisters to support myself. It amused the other students to see this crippled foreigner trying to negotiate the stairs and to find out that he was studying tai-chi, especially as everyone else was on an athletics scholarship.

I do not recommend this amount of training in the early stages: nice and easy does it, but my time was limited. I had travelled thousands of miles to study and I wanted to make use of every available moment. Gradually, my legs adjusted to the increased workload and I ceased to be an embarrassment, at least on the stairs!

Mr Mun was about forty-four years old, 6 feet tall, with a full head of grey hair. He performed the tai-chi with a smooth athletic grace that made me all the more enthusiastic to study his methods and emulate his style. His wife was from the famed Chen village where tai-chi originated, and she too held a post as instructor of tai-chi at the institute.

All wu-shu students at the institute are required to study 24-step and 48-step tai-chi, Chen style tai-chi, xing-yi and ba-gua, along with the more energetic forms and weapons. The students remain at the college for four years and eventually are sent out to various provinces to teach sports and wu-shu, unless chosen for the national team and given the opportunity to travel abroad representing China.

In all Chinese skills there are secrets to success and these are easily overlooked or underconsidered by the student. Often knowledge is imparted only when the student asks the right question at the right time. Mr Mun pointed out many elements that gave me a better understanding. I was now learning the 24-step simplified tai-chi and many of my accumulated bad habits slipped away. I began to feel great benefit from practice, improved strength and relaxation.

I also studied tai-chi sword with Mr Cho, a graduate of the college, who pointed out the principles of the sword and where the 'blade areas', which are functional, are located.

In my early days at the institute, afternoon practice coincided with the lunchtime of a young kitchen hand, who was about nineteen years old. Every day whilst I was being taught by Mr Mun, the kitchen hand would stand about 5 yards behind and follow the instruction. At first I thought he was cheeky, but soon I grew used to him, and not infrequently, when my mind went blank, he was useful. If I was making a wrong movement he would quietly hiss to me and I would correct my position.

In Chinese history there are many legends about servants who have observed the martial arts being practised and become proficient, and as the martial arts contain many legends in this area, and as he didn't disturb Mr Mun, he was allowed to remain. Occasionally Mr Mun would mutter something to him about keeping quiet, but he was allowed to continue watching and benefitting from this private lesson and he became a silent training partner. When his kitchen duties kept him away, I missed him.

It was apparent that he had had no previous training in tai-chi, but he progressed quickly.

I never cease to be amazed by the physical skills of the Chinese, the relaxed way in which they move and their high level of coordination. Compare the dexterity of a three-year-old Chinese child, who already can use chopsticks, with that of a European child of the same age.

I redoubled my efforts to study, but then remembering my experience many years earlier in Singapore, I let go. The learning process became more relaxed.

I spent about two months at the institute, undergoing the most intensive training I have ever experienced, I returned a couple of years later for corrections on my form and found that during my absence thousands of people from all over the world had visited to study tai-chi and other skills. Some of the teachers I watched on my second visit had only been students on my first.

I wondered where my young kitchen worker had gone, but it is easy to get lost amongst 1,100,000,000 people.

I feel fortunate to have found good teachers who have enriched my life with their knowledge, skill and patience. It's impossible to say where the road will lead when you take the first step.

3 An Outline History of Tai-chi and Associated Martial Arts

The incursions of Japanese pirates in league with local freeboo-ters into China's rich coastal area, particularly the soft under-belly of the Shanghai region, came to a peak in the mid-sixteenth century. Though at that time, Shanghai was not yet the great cosmopolitan entrepot it was to become in the nineteenth and twentieth centuries, already this fertile area of the Yangtze delta, including Nanking (the first Ming capital), Suzhou and Hang-zhou (the southern Sung capital) was the economic and intellectual centre of China. The region was linked by the Grand Canal to Peking (the official capital just inside the Great Wall).

The shocking success of the Japanese pirates and their hit-and-run tactics against the complacent and corrupt civil adminis-tration of the Ming at last awakened the scholar-gentry's interest in things military. Even monks, claiming affinity with the Shaolin temple and armed with iron poles, were enlisting to defend the nation.

Three great commanders, Yu Dayou (1503–79), Tang Shunzhi (1507–60) and above all Qi Jiquang (1528–88) took a personal interest in training their troops in the use of weapons and in unarmed combat. Qi Jiquang's *Boxing Classic* contains illustra-tions of thirty-two postures that remained the most explicit and detailed presentation of a set of empty-handed martial arts movements published in China before the twentieth century. This *Boxing Classic* contains the movements, with their names, that lie at the heart of modern tai-chi, even if at first sight they are hard to recognize.

In 1641, Chen Wangting was appointed to head the army reserve in Wen County, Henan Province, just north of the Yellow River. During his retirement after the fall of the Ming dynasty in 1644, he devoted himself to teaching boxing, basing his techni-que on Jiquang's *Boxing Classic* and the practice of Taoist meditation following the *Yellow Court Classic*. His descendants living in the same county continued his tradition, and apparently placed equal emphasis on physical education and self-defence. There was also a tradition of broadsword and spear forms and evidence of influence from the Shaolin temple just across the

Yellow River, south of Mount Song.

In the early nineteenth century, an outsider named Yang Lu-chan (1799–1872), from (Yongnian) in Hebei Province, sold himself as an indentured servant to the Chen clan and was permitted to learn their traditional art of boxing from Chen Chang-xing. Around 1840, after his master died, Yang obtained his freedom and returned to (Yongnian).

There, at the Great Harmony Hall medicine firm founded by his late master, he taught boxing for health. Yang's landlords, the three Wu brothers, were all taught by him.

In 1852, the second brother Wu Yuxiang, visited the Chen clan in Henan on his way to see his elder brother Wu Chengqing, who had been posted to Wuyang county in southern Henan Province. After studying over a month with Chen Qingping, Wu Yuxiang joined his brother. Meanwhile Wu Chengqing had allegedly obtained a manuscript of the *Great Polarity Boxing Theory* written by one Wang Zongyue in about 1800.

On the basis of his elder brother's find, Wu Yuxiang subsequently propounded tai-chi's theory. Yang Lu-chan subsequently went to Peking, where he began the popularization of tai-chi and founded the predominant Yang style. He seems to have made use of the myth that tai-chi is 'internal boxing'.

This 'internal system' was claimed to be superior to Shaolin and made use of acupuncture point strikes, commonly referred to as *dim-mak* ('death-touch').

It should be noted that the detailed seventeenth-century descriptions by Huang Lizhou and his son of 'internal boxing', bear no resemblance either to Chen family boxing or the *Great Polarity Boxing Theory* ascribed to Wang Zongyue.

This is the first direct link between the *Great Polarity Boxing Theory* and Chen family boxing, now known as tai-chi. The elegant style and Confucian allusions in the *Theory* make one suspect that their author was a scholar rather than a boxer, possibly Wu Yuxiang himself. If so, he may have worked up some rough notes written by Wang Zongyue and enlarged them with his own first-hand experience of the Chen family tradition.

Note

Those interested in the historical origins of tai-chi and Shaolin boxing owe a great debt to two pioneer researchers: Xu Zhen and Tang Hao. Their tireless work in assembling and critically analysing original source materials succeeded in dispelling a mass of myths.

4 Great Polarity Boxing: the Theory

attributed to (Shanxi) Wang Zongyue (late eighteenth century)

This essay is the first clear exposition of the Tai-chi philosophy in terms of self-defence and body motion.

The Great Polarity without poles is born:[1]
Of negative and positive it is the mother –
In motion divided,
In stillness, joined
Without overreaching or falling short:[2]
Following contraction, proceed to extend.

When men are hard and I am soft –
It is called 'running away';
When I go along and men are turned –
It is called 'sticking'.
Move fast and the reaction is fast,
Move slowly and the reaction is slow.
Though the metamorphoses be ten thousand,
One principle pervades them.[3]

From familiarity with the moves, one gradually awakens to
    understanding power.
Free from understanding, one by stages reaches spiritual
    enlightenment.
Without long application of effort
One cannot thoroughly fathom this.

Freely draw up the crown's power,
Let the breath sink to the point beneath the navel.
Be neither one-sided nor leaning,[4]
Suddenly conceal, suddenly reveal.
Left is full, then left empty.
Right is full, then right insubstantial.

If he looks up, it's still higher,
If he looks down, it's still deeper.[5]
If he advances, draw out longer,
If he retreats, press in closer.

One feather cannot be added
A fly cannot alight,

'Men don't know me, I alone know men',[6]
The irresistibility of the hero's progress
Is surely entirely achieved through this.[7]

This skill has many side schools.
Although each one has its distinctive postures,
As a rule they don't go beyond strong oppressing weak.
Slow yielding to fast.
Have-force beating lack-force and
Hands-slow yielding to hands-fast
Is all from innate, natural ability,
Not connected with effort of study.

Refer to the phrase: 'Four ounces deflect a thousand pounds'[8]
This is clearly not force's victory.
Regard the image of the old man able to hold off a multitude –
How could this be accomplished?

Stand like a level balance,
Lively as a carriage wheel –
Depress one side and the other follows.
When both are weighted they are impeded.

Every time I see one of several years' pure practice
Unable to manoeuvre and adapt,
Invariably causing himself by men to be controlled,
It is because the fault of double-weighting has not been realized.

Tai-chi

To avoid this fault, one must know negative and positive:
'Sticking' is 'running', 'running' is 'sticking'.
Negative does not leave positive.
Positive does not leave negative.[9]
When positive and negative complement each other,
This then is understanding power.

After understanding power,
The more practice – the more skill.
Quietly learning and experimenting,
One gradually arrives at following what the heart desires.[10]

Its root is to discard self and follow men:
Many mistakenly discard the near and seek afar.[11]
This is known as being out by a hair's breadth
And going wrong by a thousand miles.[12]
Students cannot but carefully distinguish.[13]
This is the theory.

Notes

1. Zhou Dunji (d. 1073): 'Without poles and so the Great Polarity'. The Grand Polarity gives birth to negative and positive.
2. Confucius Analects XI: 'Overreaching is like falling short.'
3. Analects IV: 'My way has One that pervades it.'
4. Document Classic: The Great Plan 'Without one-sidedness or partisanship.' Zhu Xi (1130–1200) commentary on the Central Mean (Zhongyong): 'Neither one-sided nor leaning/Without over-reaching or falling short.'
5. Analects IX: 'Look up and it is still higher, bore into it and it is still harder.'
6. Analects I: 'I don't worry about men not knowing me, I worry about not knowing men.'
7. 'A hero, whichever way he turns, is irresistible.'
8. 'Four ounces deflect a thousand pounds' is the only phrase in the tai-chi Theory which is also found in Chen family boxing, where it occurs in the couplet 'Let him with gigantic force come to strike me, I pull in motion four ounces to deflect a thousand pounds'. This concept is also claimed by the Shaolin tradition.
9. Zhou Zi Quanshu (1757): 'Negative and positive do not leave each other.' Hu Xu (d. 1736).
10. Analects II: 'At seventy I followed what my heart desired and did not transgress the rules.'
11. Documents Classic; Great Yu's Council: 'Examine the multitude, Discard the self and follow men'. Mencius: Gongsun Chou (a): 'Discard the self and follow men'.
12. Han History: *Biography of Sima Qian*: 'out by a hair's breadth, wrong by a thousand miles'.
13. Later Han History: *Biography of Zang Gong* (XVIII): 'Those who discard the near and scheme for the far, labour without result. Those who discard the far and scheme for the near, are at ease and, attain their end.'

5 Simplified 24-step Tai-chi

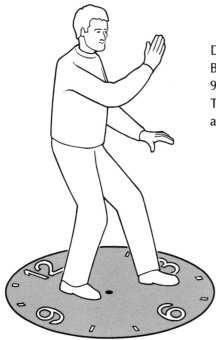

Directions are given in terms of the 12 hours of the clock.
Begin by facing 12 o'clock, with 6 o'clock behind you,
9 o'clock at your left and 3 o'clock at your right.
Thus a turn to 1 o'clock is one of 30° to the right,
and a turn to 1-2 o'clock is one of 45°.

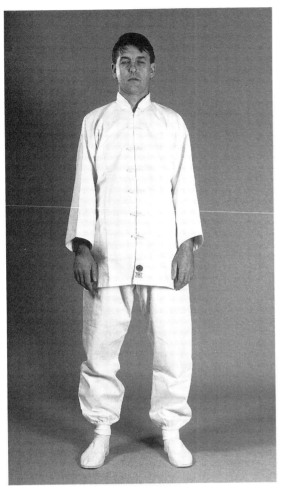

Fig. 1

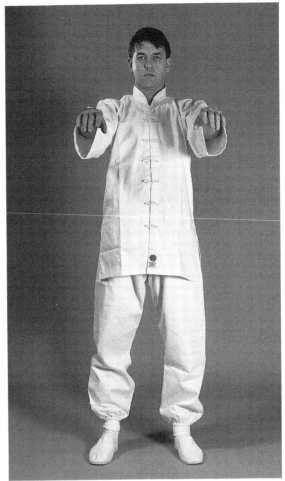

Fig. 2

SERIES I

Form 1   Commencing Form

1 Stand naturally upright with feet shoulder-width apart, toes pointing forward, arms hanging naturally and hands at your sides. Look forward. (Fig. 1)

Points to remember: Hold head and neck erect, with chin drawn slightly inward. Do not protrude chest or draw abdomen in. Be relaxed but alert and concentrating.

2 Raise arms slowly forward and upward to shoulder level with palms facing downward. (Figs. 2–3)

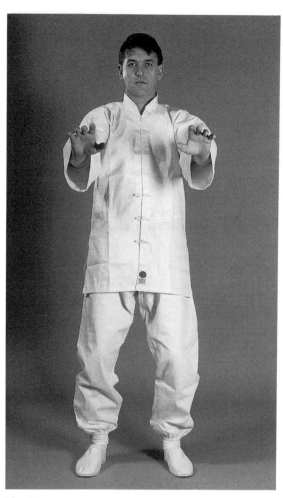

Fig. 3

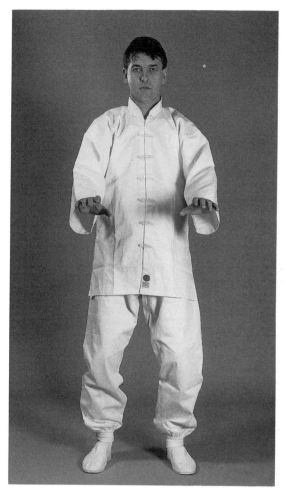

Fig. 4

3 Keeping torso erect, bend knees while pressing palms down gently, with elbows dropping towards knees. Look forward. (Fig. 4)

Points to remember: Hold shoulders and elbows down. Fingers are slightly bent. Weight is equally distributed on both legs. While bending knees, keep waist loose and relaxed and buttocks slightly pulled in. The lowering of arms should coordinate with the bending of knees.

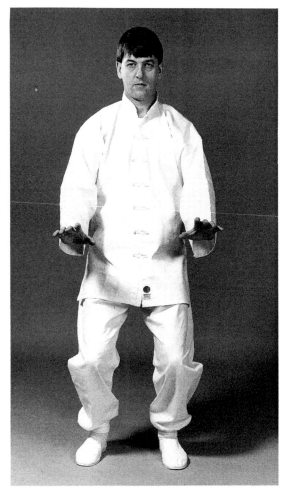

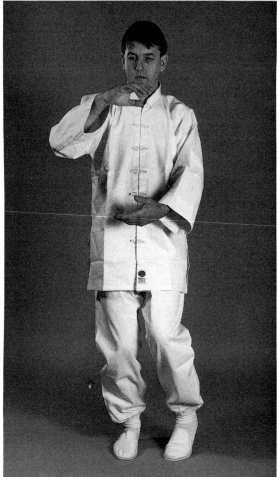

Fig. 5   **Fig. 6**

SERIES I

Form 2 Part the Wild Horse's Mane on Both Sides

1 Turn torso slightly to the right (1 o'clock) and shift weight on to right leg. Raise right hand until forearm lies horizontally in front of right part of chest, while left hand moves in a downward arc until it comes under right hand, palms facing each other as if holding a ball (henceforth referred to as a 'holdball gesture'). Close left foot to the side of the right and rest its toes on floor. Look at right hand. (Figs. 5–6)

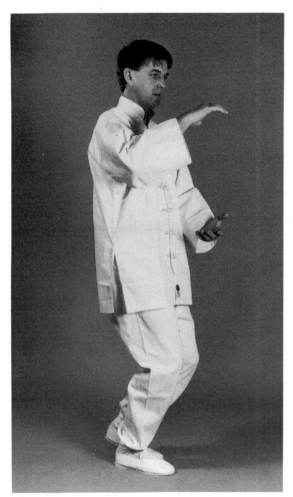

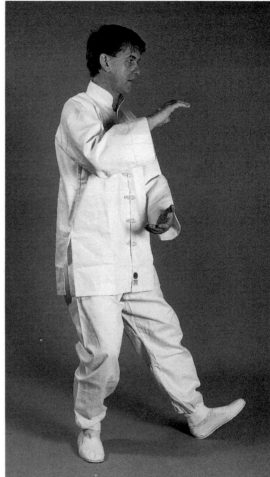

Fig. 7

Fig. 8

2 Turn body to the left (10 o'clock) while left foot takes a step forward towards 8–9 o'clock, bending knee and shifting weight on to left leg, and right leg straightens with heel pressing down on floor to form a left 'bow step.' At the same time as you turn your body slightly leftward, gradually raise left forearm obliquely to eye level with palm facing obliquely upward and elbow slightly bent, and lower right hand to the side of right hip with palm facing downward and fingers pointing forward. *Look at left hand.* (Figs. 7–9)

31

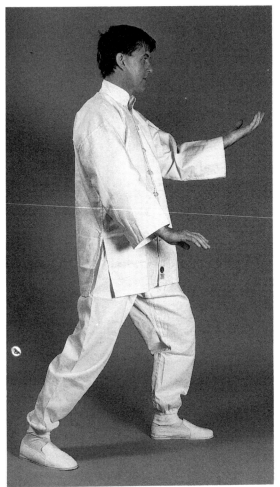

Fig. 9

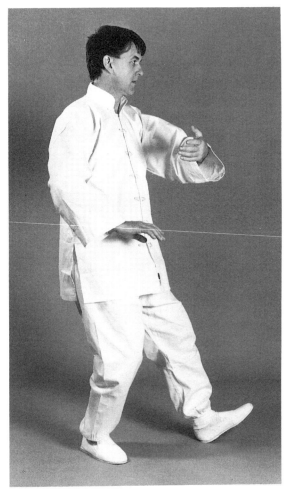

Fig. 10

3 'Sit back' slowly – move torso backward as if ready to take a seat – and shift weight on to right leg. Raise toes of left foot slightly and turn them outward before placing the foot flat on floor. Then bend left leg and turn body to the left (5 o'clock), shifting weight back again on to left leg. Make a hold-ball gesture in front of left part of chest, left hand on top. Then draw right foot forward to side of left foot and rest its toes on floor. Look at left hand. (Figs. 10–12)

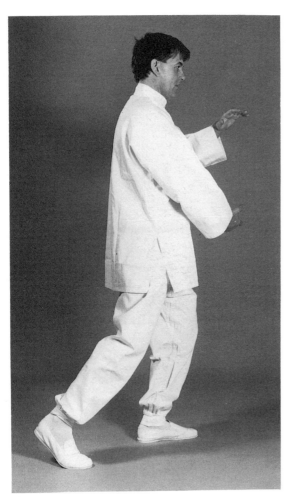

Fig. 11

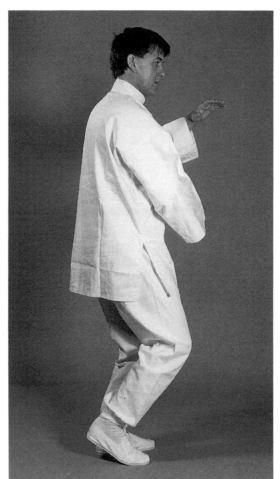

Fig. 12

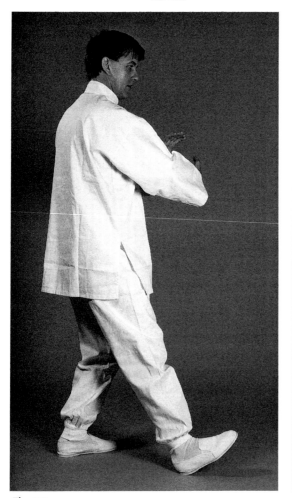

Fig. 13

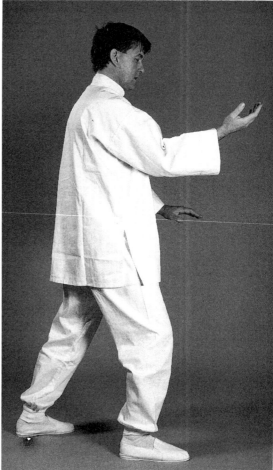

Fig. 14

4   Take a right bow step by moving right foot a step towards 9–10 o'clock, straightening left leg with heel pressing down on floor and bending right leg at knee. At the same time, turn body to the right (8 o'clock), gradually raise right hand obliquely upward to eye level with palm facing obliquely upward and elbows slightly bent, and press left hand down to the side of left hip with palm facing downward and fingers pointing forward. Look at right hand. (Figs. 13–14)

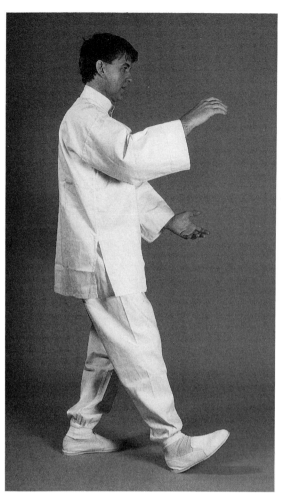

Fig. 15

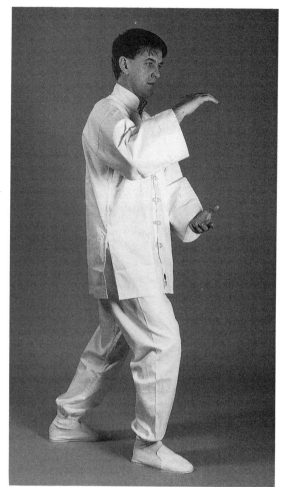

Fig. 16

5 Repeat movements in 3 above, reversing 'right' and 'left.' (Figs. 15–17)

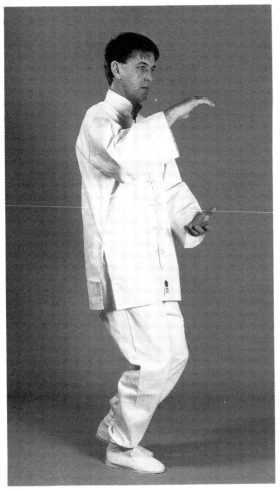

Fig. 17

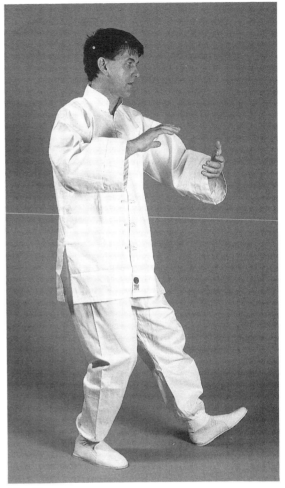

Fig. 18

6 Repeat movements in 4, reversing 'right' and 'left'. (Figs. 18–19)

Points to remember: Hold torso erect and keep chest relaxed. Arms should move in an arc. Keep arms from being fully stretched when you separate hands. In turning body, waist serves as the axis. Tempo of movement in taking bow steps and in separating hands must be even and synchronized. When stepping forward, place your foot slowly in position, heel coming down first. Knee of front leg should not go beyond toes, which should point forward; the rear leg should straighten backward a bit and let the rear foot form an

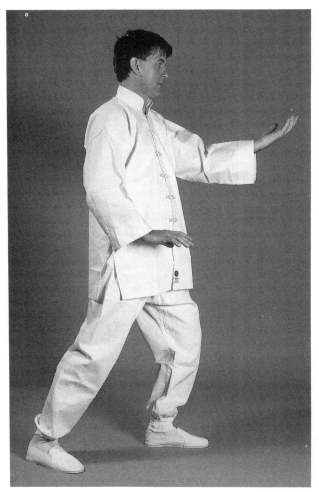

Fig. 19

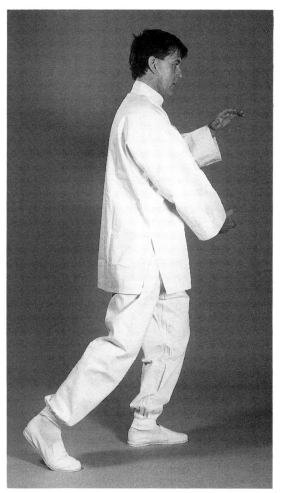

Fig. 20

angle of 45–60 degrees with the front one. Heels should not be in a straight line, the transverse distance between them being 10–30 cm. Face 9 o'clock in the final position.

SERIES I

Form 3   The White Crane Spreads Its Wings

1 Turn torso slightly to the left (8 o'clock). Make a hold-ball gesture in front of left part of chest, left hand on top. Look at left hand. (Fig. 20)

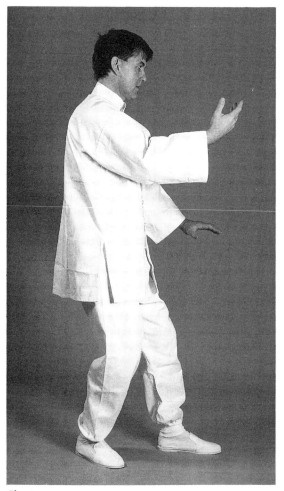

Fig. 21

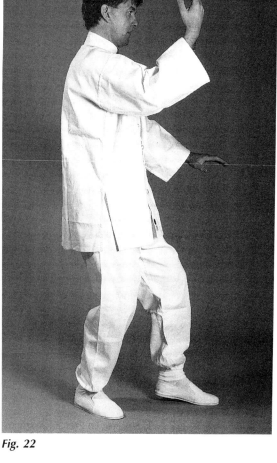

Fig. 22

2 Draw right foot half a step towards left foot and then sit back. Turn torso slightly to the right (10 o'clock). Look at right hand with weight on right leg, move left foot slightly forward and rest its toes lightly on floor. (You have now taken a left 'empty step.') At the same time, turn torso slightly to the left (9 o'clock), and raise right hand until it is in front of right temple, palm turned inward, while left hand moves downward until it stops in front of left hip, palm turned downward and fingers pointing forward. Look straight ahead. (Figs. 21–22)

Points to remember: Do not thrust chest forward. Arms should be rounded when they move up or down. Bend left leg slightly at knee. Shift of weight backwards should be coordinated with the raising of right hand. Face 9 o'clock in the final position.

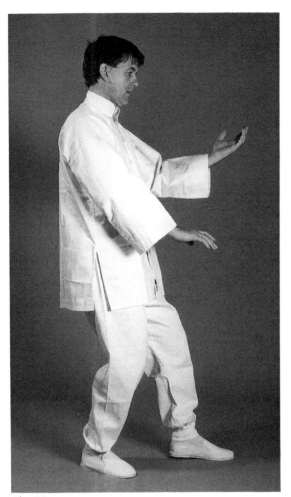

Fig. 23

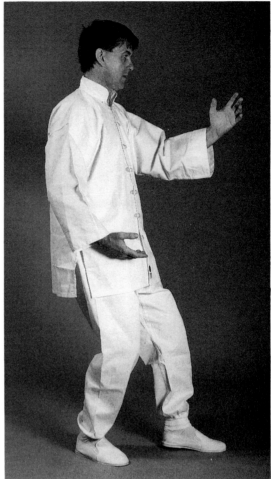

Fig. 24

SERIES II

Form 4   Brush Knee and Twist Step on Both Sides

1 Turn torso slightly to the left (8 o'clock); right hand moves downward while left hand moves upward. Turn torso to the right (11 o'clock), right hand circles past abdomen and then upward to ear level with arm slightly bent and palm facing obliquely upward, while left hand moves first in an upward and then in a downward curve, stopping before right part of chest, palm facing obliquely downward. Look at right hand. (Figs. 23–25)

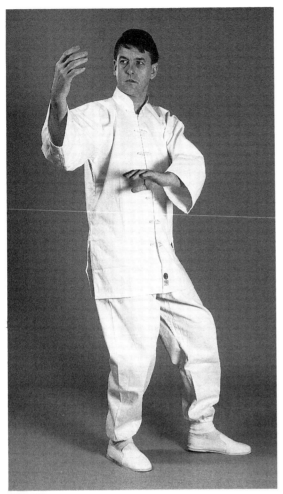

Fig. 25

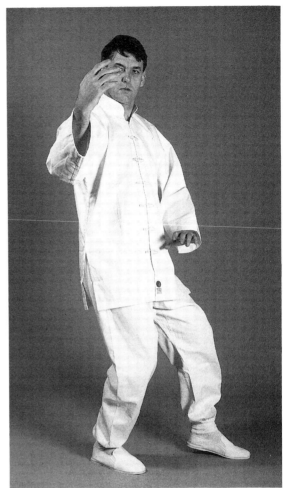

Fig. 26

2 Turn torso to the left (9 o'clock). Left foot takes a step forward towards 8 o'clock to form a left bow step. At the same time, right hand draws leftward past right ear and, following body turn, pushes forward at nose level with palm facing forward, while left hand drops and circles around left knee to stop beside left hip with palm facing downward. Look at fingers of right hand. (Figs. 26–27)

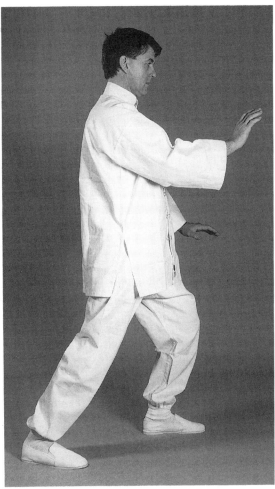

Fig. 27

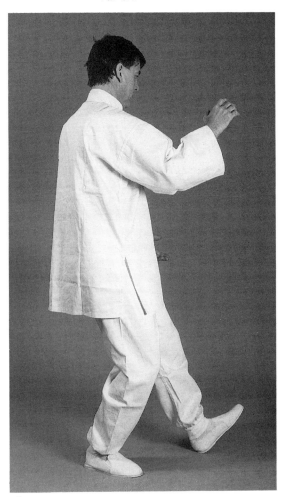

Fig. 28

3 Sit back with right knee slowly bent, shifting weight on to right leg. Raise toes of left foot and turn them a bit outward before placing foot flat on floor. Then bend the leg slowly. Turn body to the left (7 o'clock) and shift weight on to left leg. Bring right foot forward to the side of left foot and rest its toes on floor. At the same time, turn left palm up and, with elbow slightly bent, move left hand sideways and up to shoulder level, palm turning obliquely upward, while right hand, following body turn, makes an arc upward and then downward to the left, stopping in front of left part of chest, palm facing obliquely downward. Look at left hand. (Figs. 28–30)

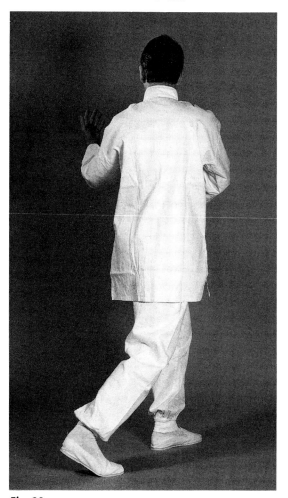

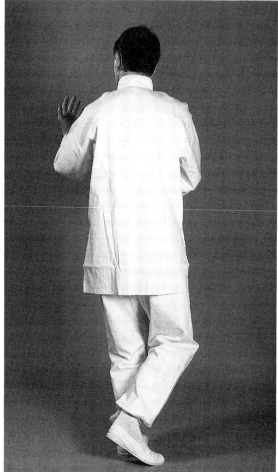

Fig. 29

Fig. 30

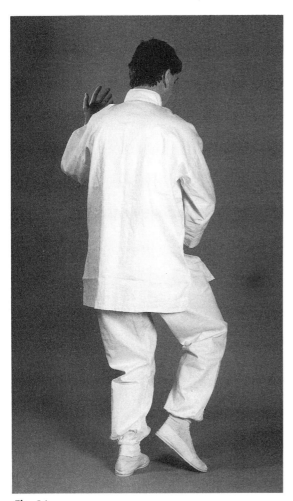

Fig. 31

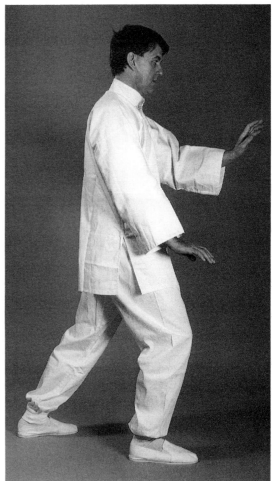

Fig. 32

4 Repeat movements in 2, reversing 'right' and 'left.' (Figs. 31–32)

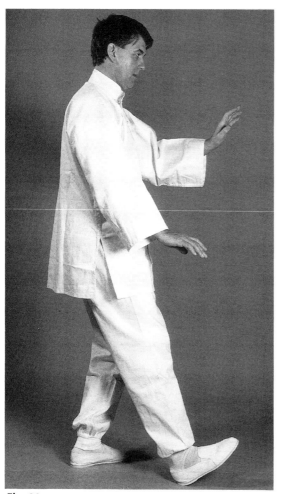

Fig. 33

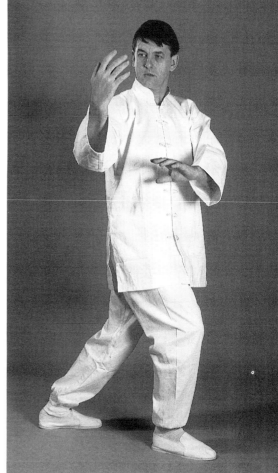

Fig. 34

5 Repeat movements in 3, reversing 'right' and 'left.' (Figs. 33–35)

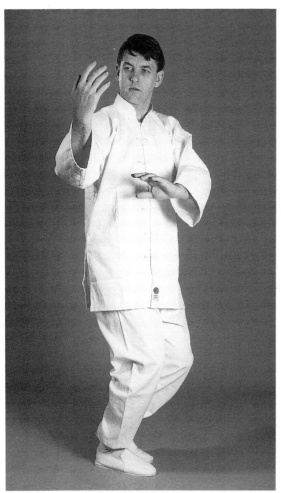

Fig. 35

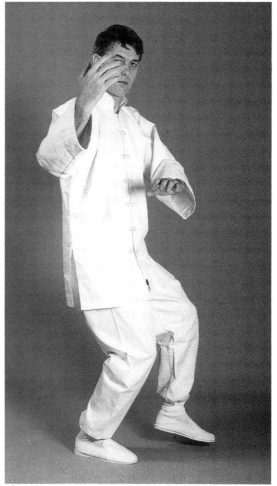

Fig. 36

6 Repeat movements in 2. (Figs. 36–37)

Points to remember: Keep torso erect while pushing hands forward. Waist and hips should be relaxed. When pushing palm forward, hold shoulders and elbows down and keep waist relaxed. Movements of palm should be coordinated with those of waist and leg. Transverse distance between heels should not be less than 30 cm. Face 9 o'clock in the final position.

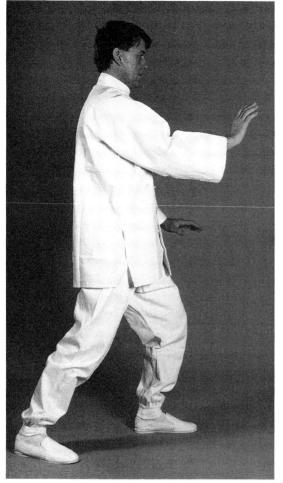

Fig. 37

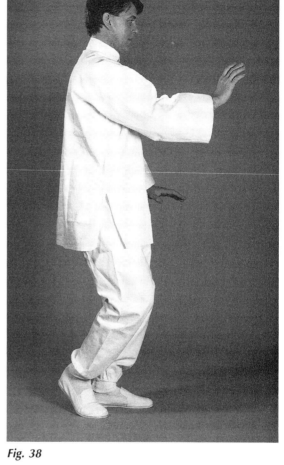

Fig. 38

SERIES II

Form 5   Hand Strums the Lute

Move right foot half a step forward towards left heel. Sit back and turn torso slightly to the right (10–11 o'clock), shifting weight on to right leg. Raise left foot and place it slightly forward, heel coming down on floor and knee bent a little to form a left empty step. Meanwhile, raise left hand in a curve to nose-tip level, with palm facing towards the right and elbow slightly bent. Right hand moves downward until it reaches the inside of left elbow, palm facing to the left. Look at

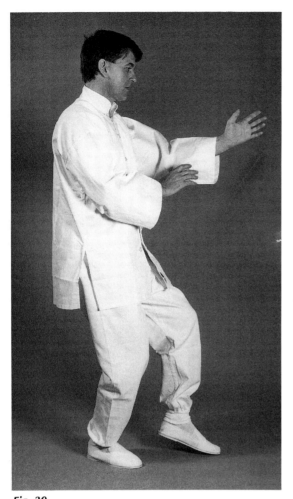

Fig. 39

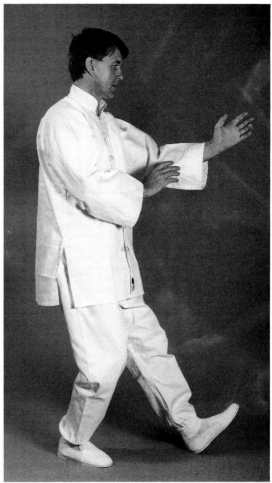

Fig. 40

forefinger of left hand. (Figs. 38–40)

5 Turn torso slightly to the left (10 o'clock). Bend right arm and place right hand inside left wrist. Turn torso a little further to the left (9 o'clock). Press both hands slowly forward with right palm facing forward and left palm inward, left arm being rounded. Meanwhile, shift weight slowly on to left leg to form a bow step. Look at left wrist. (Figs. 61–62)

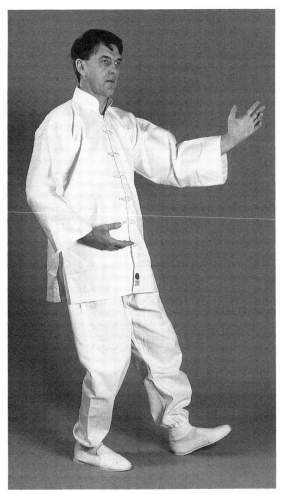

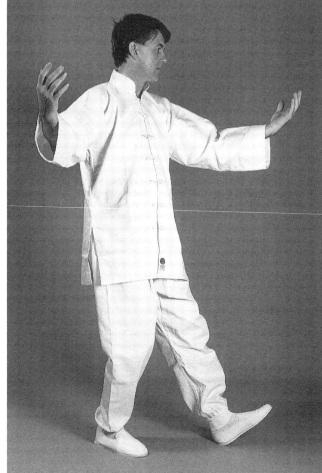

Fig. 41   **Fig. 42**

SERIES II

Form 6   *Step Back and Whirl Arms on Both Sides*

1 Turn torso slightly to the right (11–12 o'clock). Right hand makes a semicircle past abdomen and upward to shoulder level with palm facing upward and arm slightly bent. Turn left palm up and place toes of left foot on floor. First look to the right as body turns in that direction, then turn around to look ahead at left hand. (Figs. 41–42)

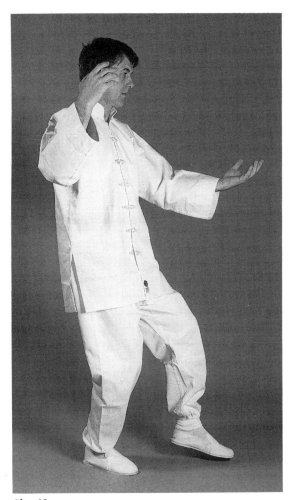

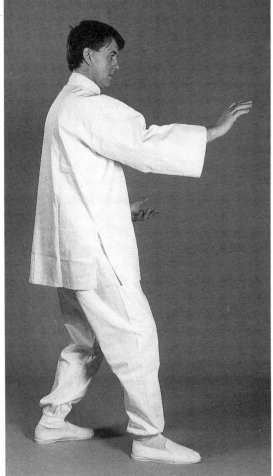

Fig. 43

Fig. 44

2 Bend right arm and draw hand past the ear before pushing it ahead with palm facing forward. Pull left hand back until it is beside waist, palm facing upward. At the same time, raise left foot lightly and take a step backward toward 3–4 o'clock, placing it slowly in position from toes to heel. Turn body to the left (8 o'clock) and shift weight on to left leg to form a right empty step, with right foot pivoting on toes until it points forward. Look at right hand. (Figs. 43–44)

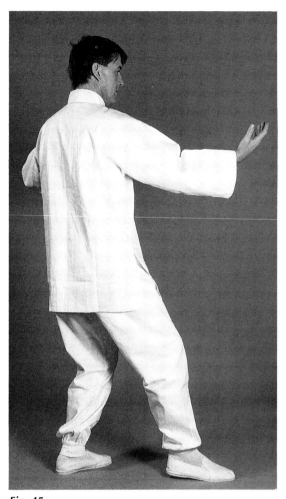

Fig. 45

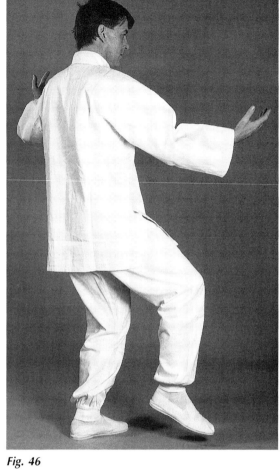

Fig. 46

3 Turn torso slightly to the left (6–7 o'clock). At the same time, carry left hand sideways and up to shoulder level, palm facing upward, while right palm is turned up. Eyes first look to the left as body turns in that direction, then turn around to look ahead at right hand. (Fig. 45)

4 Repeat movements in 2, reversing 'right' and 'left.' (Figs. 46–47)

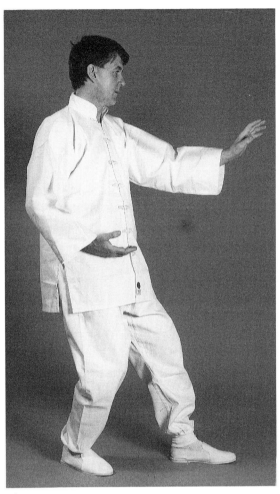

Fig. 47

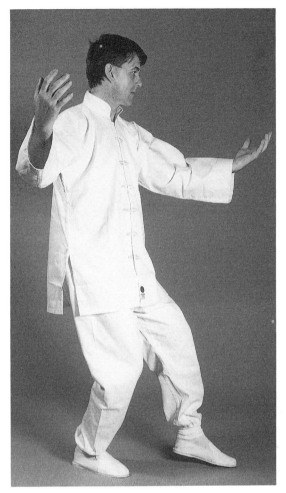

Fig. 48

5 Repeat movements in 3, reversing 'right' and 'left.' (Fig. 48)

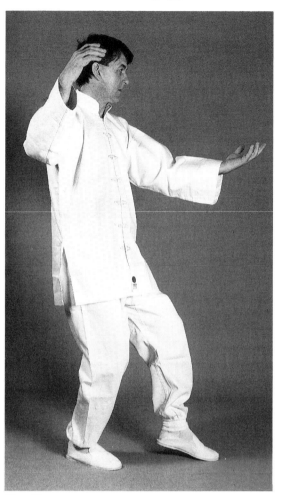

Fig. 49

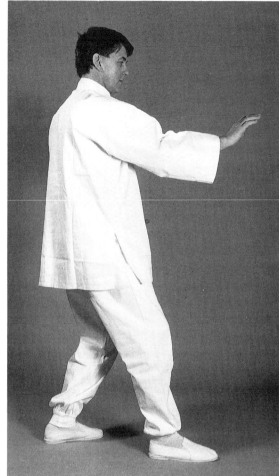

Fig. 50

6 Repeat movements in 2. (Figs. 49–50)

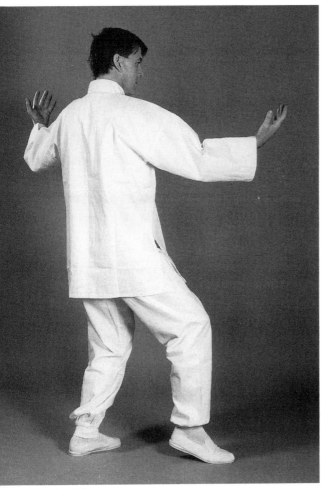

Fig. 51

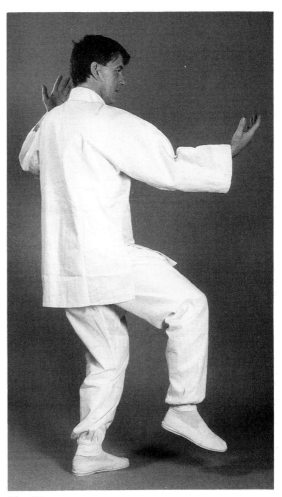

Fig. 52

7   Repeat movements in 3. (Fig. 51)

8   Repeat movements in 2, reversing 'right' and 'left.' (Figs. 52–53)

Points to remember: In pushing out or drawing back, hands should not go straight but should move in an arc. While pushing out hands, keep waist and hips relaxed. The turning of waist should be coordinated with hand movements. When stepping back, place toes down first and then slowly set the whole foot on floor. Simultaneously with body turn, front foot is turned, pivoting on toes, until it comes in line with body. Move left leg slightly towards the left, or right leg slightly towards the right, as the case may be, when taking a

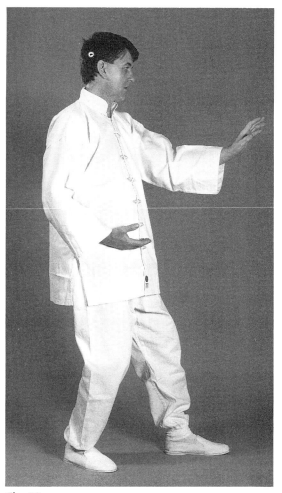

Fig. 53

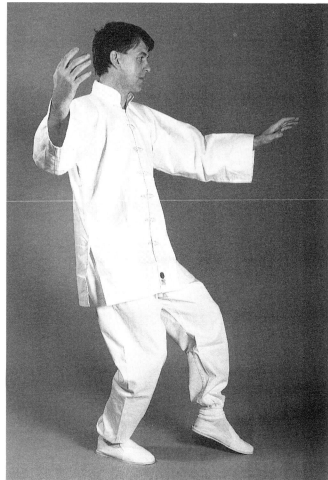

Fig. 54

step backwards, taking care not to let the feet land in a straight line. Depending on the direction of body turn, first look to the left or the right and then turn to look at the hand in front. Face 9 o'clock in the final position.

SERIES III

Form 7   *Grasp the Bird's Tail – Left Style*

1 Turn torso slightly to the right (11–12 o'clock). At the same time, carry right hand sideways and up to shoulder level, palm facing upward, while left palm is turned downward. Look at left hand. (Fig. 54)

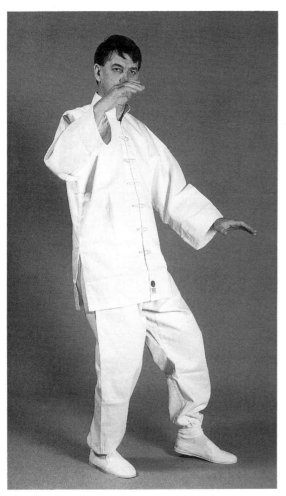

Fig. 55

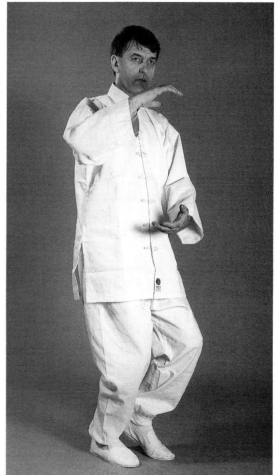

Fig. 56

2 Turn body slightly to the right (12 o'clock). Make a hold-ball gesture in front of right part of chest, right hand on top. At the same time, shift weight on to right leg, draw left foot to the side of right foot and rest its toes on floor. Look at right hand. (Figs. 55–56)

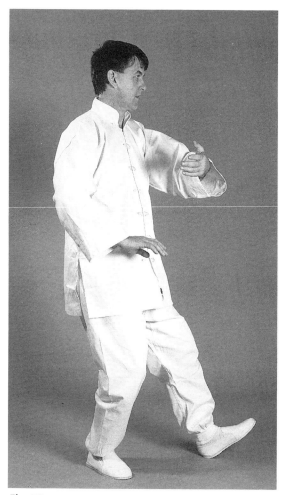

Fig. 57

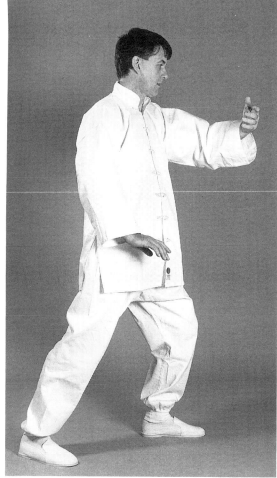

Fig. 58

3 Turn torso slightly to the left (11 o'clock). Left foot takes a step forward towards 8–9 o'clock. Turn torso a bit further to the left (10 o'clock), and bend left leg to form a bow step, with right leg naturally straightened. Meanwhile, push out the rounded left forearm at shoulder level with palm facing inward. Right hand drops slowly to the side of right hip, palm facing downward and fingers pointing forward. Look at left forearm. (Figs. 57–58)

Points to remember: Keep both arms rounded while pushing out one of them. The separation of hands, relaxing of waist and bending of leg must all be coordinated.

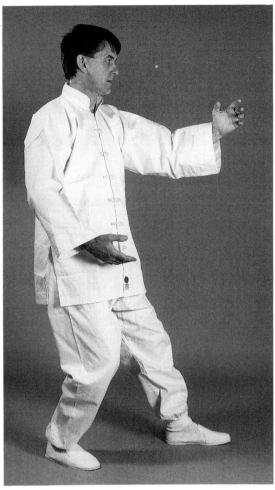

Fig. 59

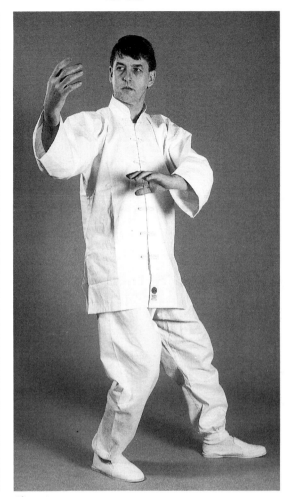

Fig. 60

4 Turn torso slightly to the left (9 o'clock) while extending left hand forward with palm turned down. Bring right hand upward, palm turning up, until it is below left forearm. Then turn torso to the right (11 o'clock) while pulling both hands down in such a way as to draw an arc before abdomen, finishing with right hand extended sideways at shoulder level, palm up, and left forearm lying across chest, palm turned inward. At the same time, shift weight on to right leg. Look at right hand. (Figs. 59–60)

Points to remember: while hands are pulled down, do not lean forward or let buttocks protrude. Arms should follow the turning of waist and move in a circular path.

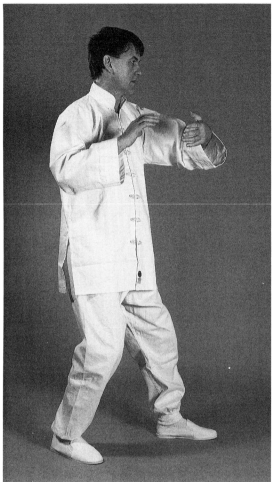

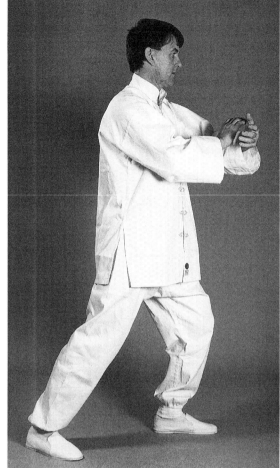

Fig. 61

Fig. 62

5 Turn torso slightly to the left (10 o'clock). Bend right arm and place right hand inside left wrist. Turn torso a little further to the left (9 o'clock). Press both hands slowly forward with right palm facing forward and left palm inward, left arm being rounded. Meanwhile, shift weight slowly on to left leg to form a bow step. Look at left wrist. (Figs. 61–62)

Points to remember: Keep torso erect when pressing hands forward; the movement of hands must be coordinated with the relaxing of waist and bending of leg.

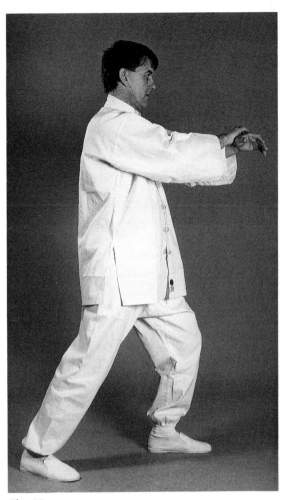

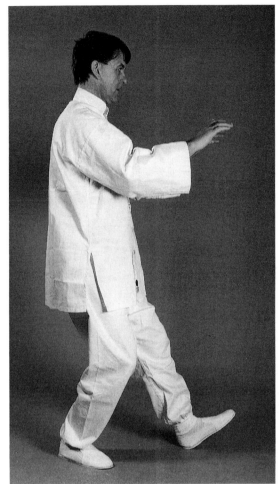

Fig. 63

Fig. 64

6 Turn both palms downward as right hand passes over left wrist and moves forward and then to the right, ending on a level with left hand. Separate hands shoulder-width apart and sit back, shifting weight on to the slightly bent right leg, with toes of left foot turned up. Draw back both hands to the front of abdomen, palms facing slightly downward to the front. Look straight ahead. (Figs. 63–65)

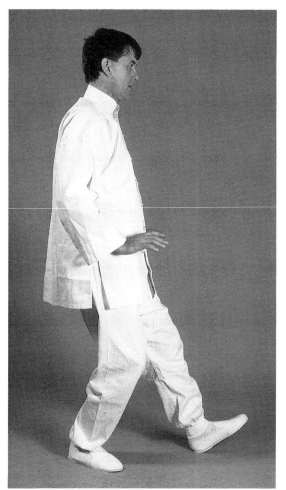

Fig. 65

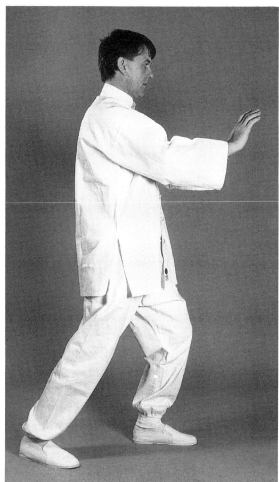

Fig. 66

7   Slowly transfer weight on to left leg while pushing hands forward and obliquely up with palms facing forward, until wrists are shoulder high. At the same time, bend left knee into a bow step. Look forward. Face 9 o'clock in the final position. (Fig. 66)

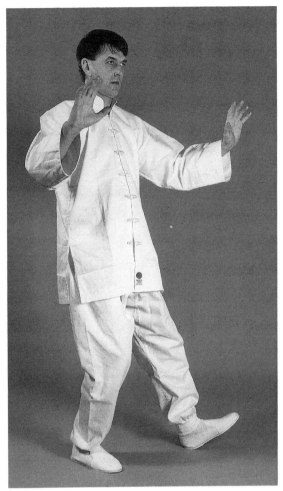

Fig. 67

Fig. 68

SERIES III

Form 8   Grasp the Bird's Tail – Right Style

1   Sit back and turn torso to the right (12 o'clock), shifting weight on to right leg and turning toes of left foot inward. Right hand makes a horizontal arc to the right, then moves downward past abdomen and upward to the left ribs, palm facing upward, forming a hold-ball gesture with left hand on top. Meanwhile, weight is shifted back on to left leg. Place right foot beside the left with heel raised. Look at left hand. (Figs. 67–70)

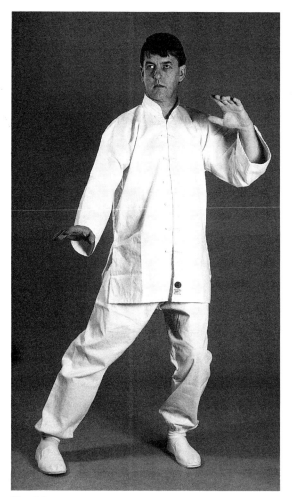

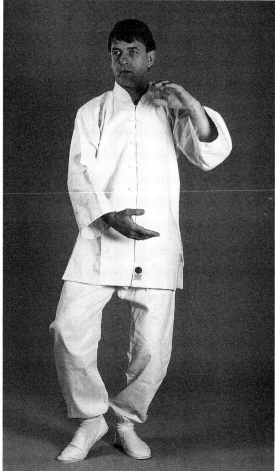

Fig. 69   *Fig. 70*

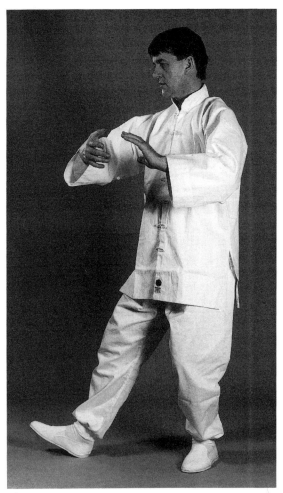

Fig. 71

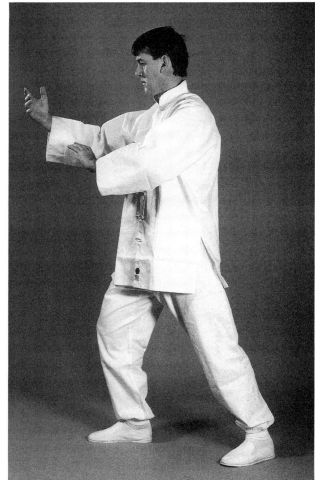

Fig. 72

2 Repeat movement in 3 of Form 7, reversing 'right' and 'left'. (Figs. 71–72)

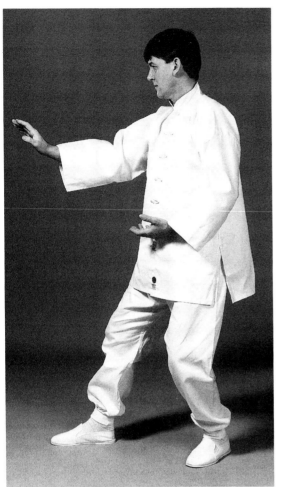

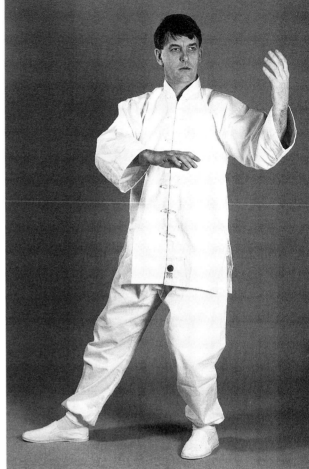

Fig. 73

Fig. 74

3 Repeat movements in 4 of Form 7, reversing 'right' and 'left'. (Figs. 73–74)

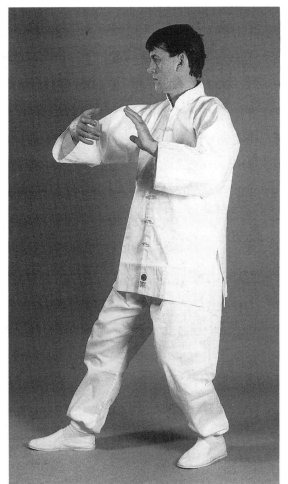

Fig. 75

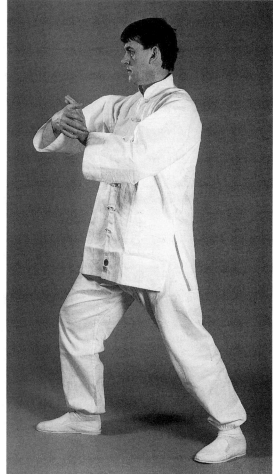

Fig. 76

4 Repeat movements in 5 of Form 7, reversing 'right' and 'left'. (Figs. 75–76)

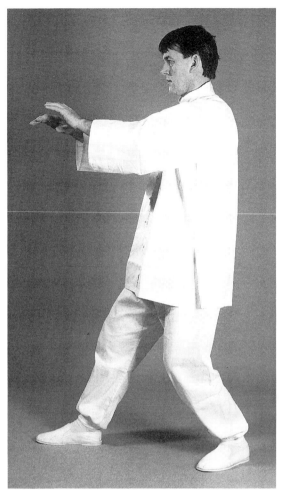

Fig. 77

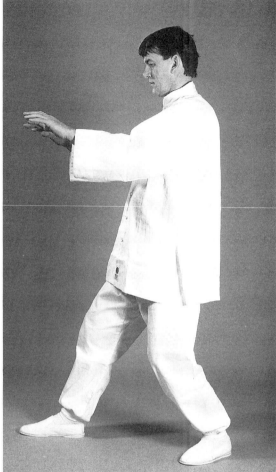

Fig. 78

5 Repeat movements in 6 of Form 7, reversing 'right' and 'left.' (Figs. 77–79)

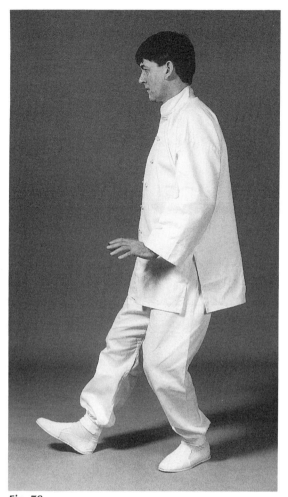

Fig. 79

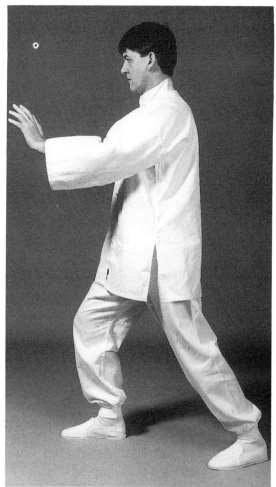

Fig. 80

6 Repeat movements in 7 of Form 7, reversing 'right' and 'left.' (Fig. 80)

Points to remember: The same as those for Form 7. Face 3 o'clock in the final position.

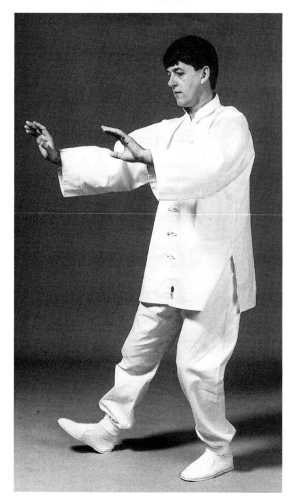

Fig. 81

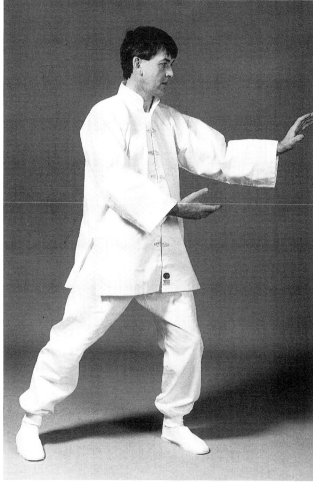

Fig. 82

SERIES IV

Form 9   Single Whip

1   Sit back and gradually shift weight on to left leg while toes of right foot are turned inward. Meanwhile, turn body to the left (11 o'clock). Move both hands leftward, left hand on top, until left arm is sideways at shoulder level, palm facing outward, and right hand is in front of left ribs, palm facing obliquely inward. Look at left hand. (Figs. 81–82)

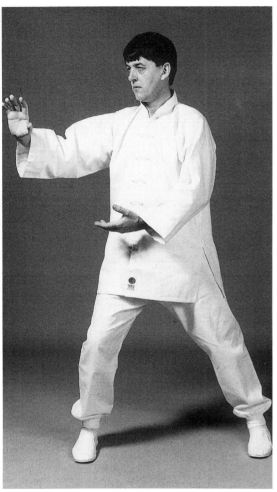

Fig. 83

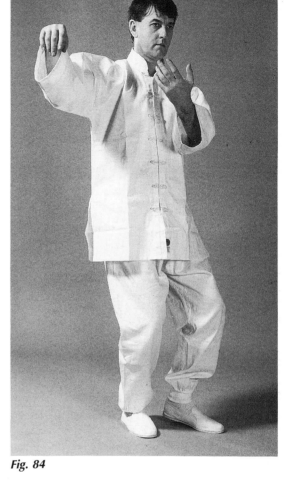

Fig. 84

2 Turn body to the right (1 o'clock), shifting weight gradually on to right leg. Draw left foot to the side of the right and rest its toes on floor. At the same time, right hand makes an arc upward and round to the right until arm is at shoulder level. With right palm now turned outward, bunch fingertips and turn them downward from wrist to form a 'hooked hand,' while left hand moves in an arc past abdomen and ends in front of right shoulder with palm facing inward. Look at left hand. (Figs. 83–84)

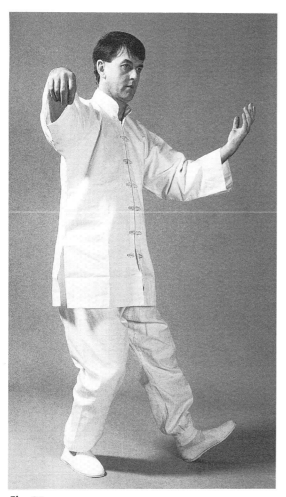

Fig. 85

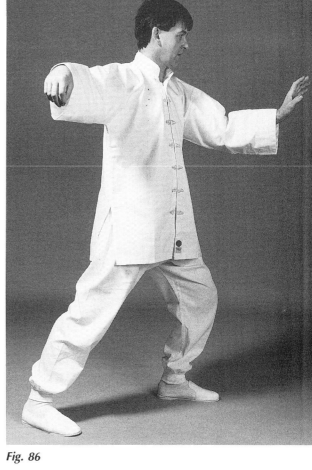

Fig. 86

3 Turn body to the left (10 o'clock) while left foot takes a step forward towards 8–9 o'clock. Bend left knee into a bow step. While shifting weight on to left leg, rotate left palm slowly and push it ahead with fingertips at eye level and elbow slightly bent. Look at left hand. (Figs. 85–86)

Points to remember: Keep torso erect and waist relaxed. Right elbow should be slightly bent downward and left elbow directly above left knee. Lower shoulders. Left palm is turned in time with the pressing forward of left hand; see to it that it is not turned too quickly or abruptly. All transitional movements must be well coordinated. Face 8–9 o'clock in the final position.

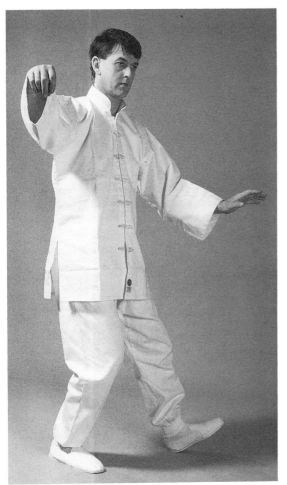

Fig. 87

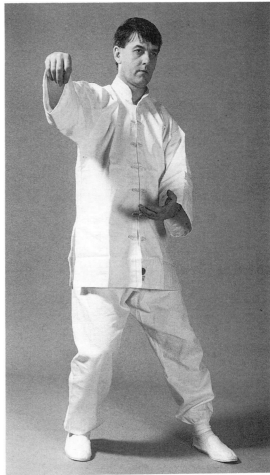

Fig. 88

SERIES IV

Form 10   Wave Hands Like Clouds – Left Style

1 Shift weight on to right leg and turn body gradually to the right (1–2 o'clock), while toes of left foot are turned inward. Left hand makes an arc past abdomen and finishes in front of right shoulder with palm turned obliquely inward. At the same time, open right hand and turn palm outward. Look at left hand. (Figs. 87–89)

71

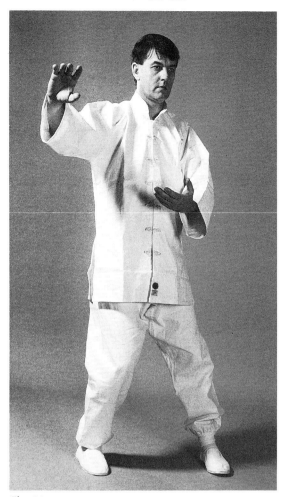

Fig. 89

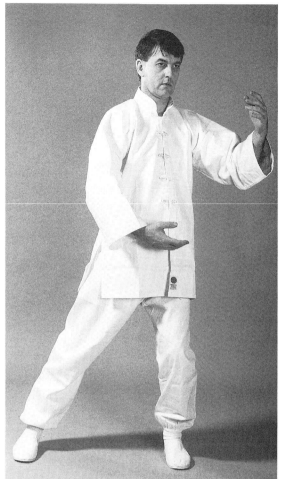

Fig. 90

2 Turn torso gradually to the left (10–11 o'clock), shifting weight on to left leg. Left hand makes an arc past the face with palm turned slowly outward. Right hand makes an arc past abdomen and then upward to left shoulder with palm turned obliquely inward. Meanwhile, bring right foot to the side of the left so that feet are parallel and 10–20 cm. apart. Look at right hand. (Figs. 90–91)

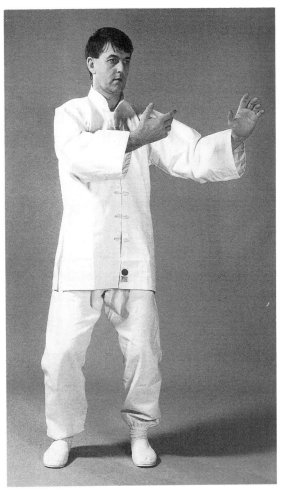

Fig. 91

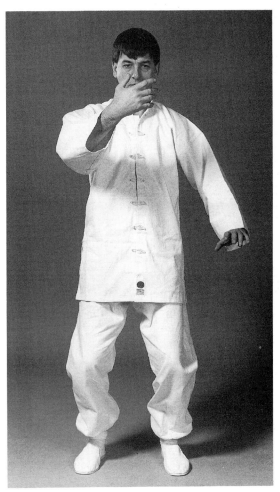

Fig. 92

3 Turn torso gradually to the right (1–2 o'clock), shifting weight on to right leg. Right hand continues to move to the right side past the face, palm turned outward, while left hand makes an arc past abdomen and upward to shoulder level with palm turned obliquely inward. Left foot then takes a side step. Look at left hand. (Figs. 92–94)

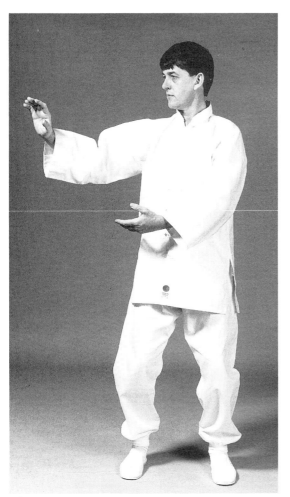

Fig. 93

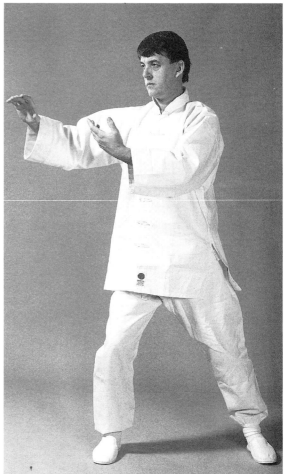

Fig. 94

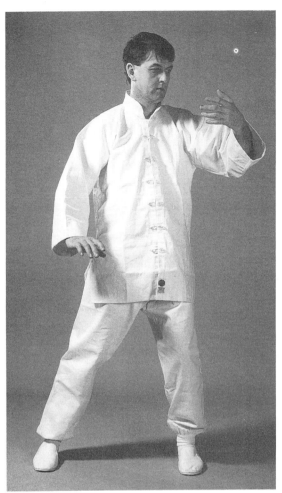

Fig. 95

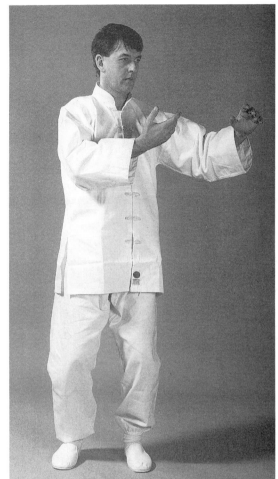

Fig. 96

4 Repeat movements in 2. (Figs. 95–96)

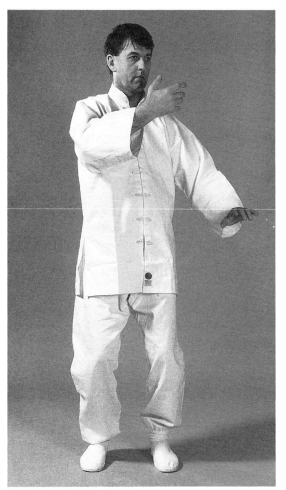

Fig. 97

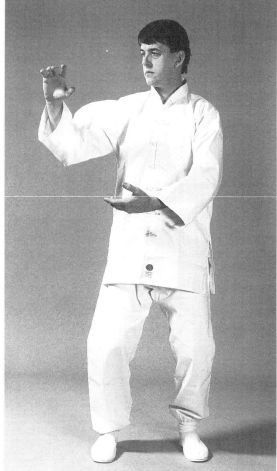

Fig. 98

5 Repeat movements in 3. (Figs. 97–99)

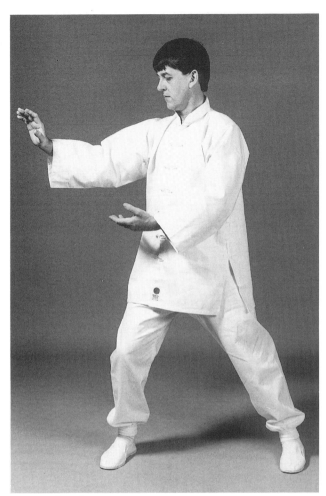

Fig. 99

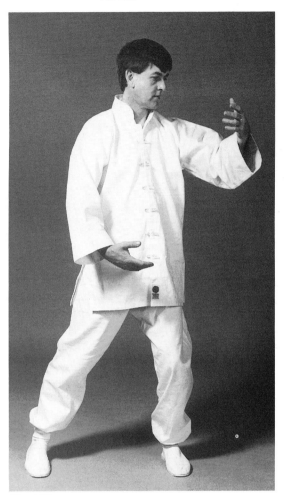

Fig. 100

6   Repeat movements in 2. (Figs. 100–101)

Points to remember: Lumbar spine serves as the axis for body turns. Keep waist and hips relaxed and avoid a sudden rise or fall of body position. Movement of arms should be natural and circular and should follow that of waist. The pace must be slow and even. Keep your balance when moving lower limbs. Eyes should follow the hand when it moves past the face. Body in the final position faces 10–11 o'clock.

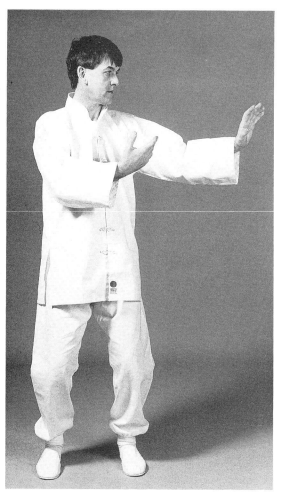

Fig. 101

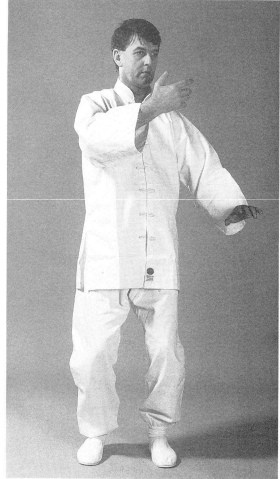

Fig. 102

SERIES IV

Form 11   Single Whip

1   Turn torso to the right (1 o'clock). At the same time, right hand moves towards the right side and forms a hooked hand at a point a little higher than shoulder level, while left hand makes an arc past abdomen and then upward to right shoulder with palm turned inward. Weight is shifted on to right leg, while toes of left foot rest on floor. Look at left hand. (Figs. 102–104)

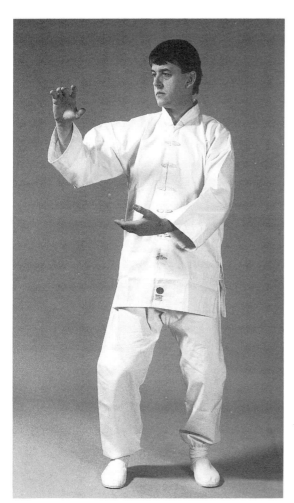

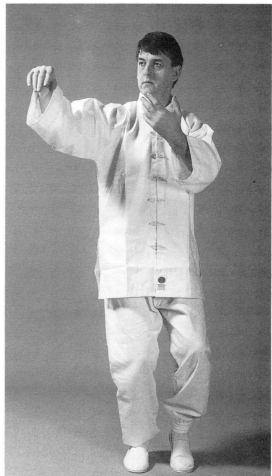

Fig. 103

Fig. 104

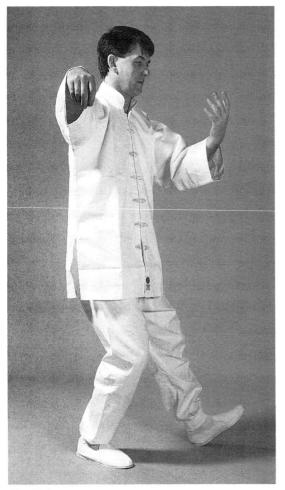

Fig. 105

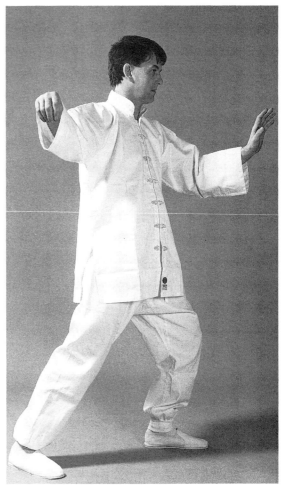

Fig. 106

2 Movements are the same as in 3 of Form 9. (Figs. 105–106)

Points to remember: The same as those for Form 9. Face 8–9 o'clock in the final position.

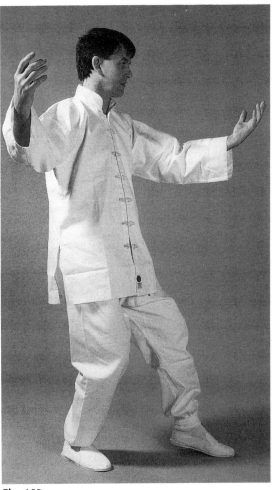

Fig. 107

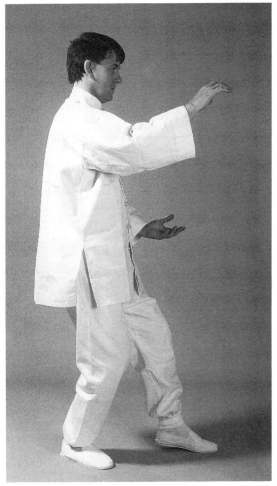

Fig. 108

SERIES V

Form 12   High Pat on Horse

1   Right foot takes half a step forward; then shift weight on to right leg. Open right hand and turn both palms upward with elbows slightly bent, while body turns slightly to the right (10–11 o'clock) with left heel gradually raised to form an empty step. Look forward to the left. (Fig 107)

2   Turn body slightly to the left (9 o'clock); draw right hand past right ear and push it forward with palm facing forward and fingers pointing up at eye level. Lower left hand until it comes in front of left hip, palm still facing upward. Meanwhile, bring left foot slightly forward with toes on floor. Look at right hand. (Fig. 108)

Points to remember: Hold torso erect and relaxed. Hold shoulders low and bend right elbow slightly downward. Do not let body rise or fall when shifting weight on to right leg. Face 9 o'clock in the final position.

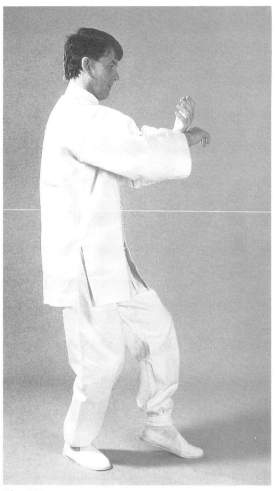

Fig. 109

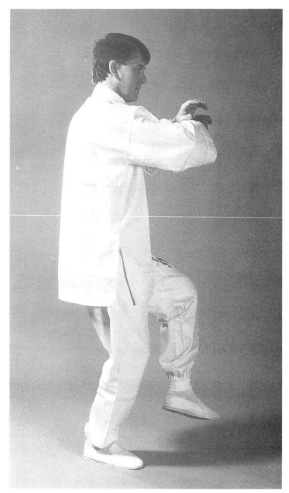

Fig. 110

SERIES V

Form 13   Kick with Right Heel

1   Cross hands by extending left hand, palm upward, on to the back of right wrist. Then hands separate, each making an arc downward on one side with palm turned obliquely downward. Meanwhile, left foot is raised to make a step forward towards 8 o'clock, forming a left bow step, toes turned slightly outward. Look straight forward. (Figs. 109–111)

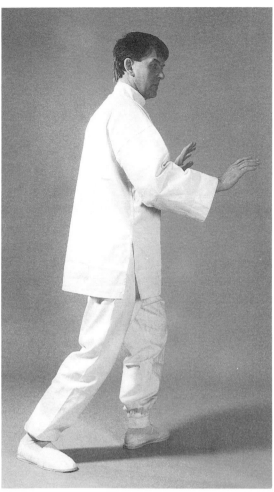

Fig. 111

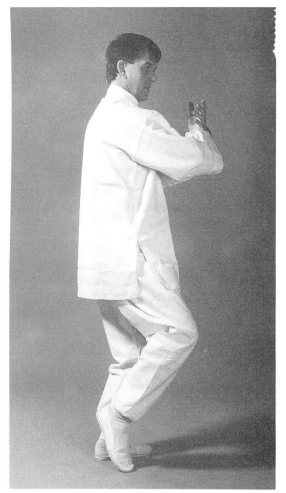

Fig. 112

2 Both hands continue to circle outward and then inward and upward until they cross in front of chest, both palms turned inward, with the back of left hand against the inside of right wrist. At the same time, bring right foot to the side of the left and rest its toes on floor. Look forward to the right. (Fig. 112)

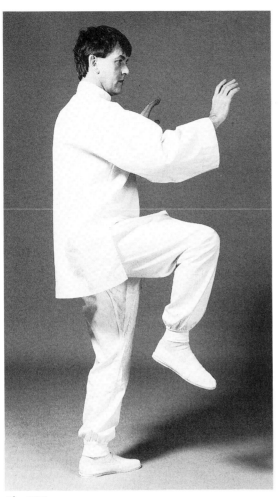

Fig. 113

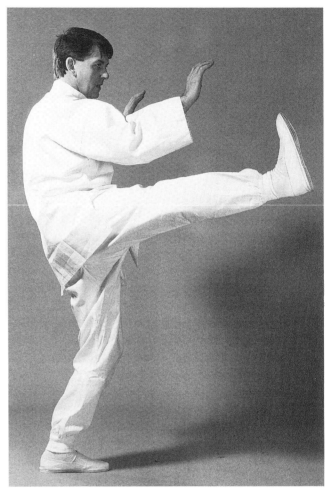

Fig. 114

3 Separate hands, extending them sideways at shoulder level, with elbows slightly bent and palms turned outward. At the same time, raise right leg, bent at knee, and thrust foot gradually forward towards 10 o'clock. Look at right hand. (Figs. 113–114)

Points to remember: Keep your balance. Wrists are level with shoulders when hands are separated. Left leg is lightly bent when right foot kicks forward, and the force of the kick should be from the heel, with upturned toes pointing slightly inward. The separation of hands should coordinate with the kick. Right arm is parallel with right leg. Face 9 o'clock in the final position.

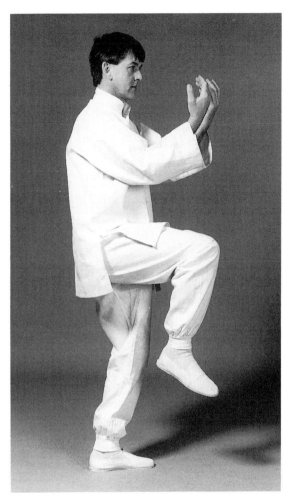

Fig. 115

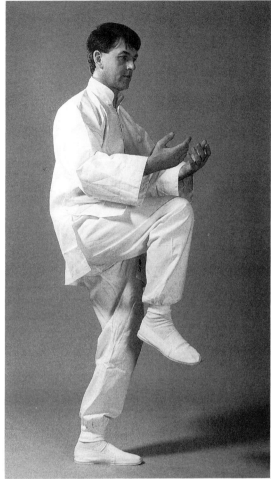

Fig. 116

SERIES V

Form 14   Strike Opponent's Ears with Both Fists

1 Pull back right foot and keep it suspended by bending knee so that thigh is level. Move left hand up and forward, then down to the side of right hand in front of chest, turning both palms up. Both hands make a circular movement downward, dropping on both sides of right knee. Look straight forward. (Figs. 115–116)

85

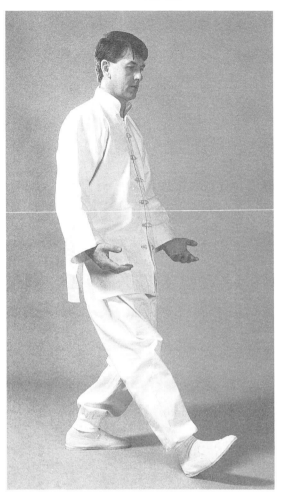

Fig. 117

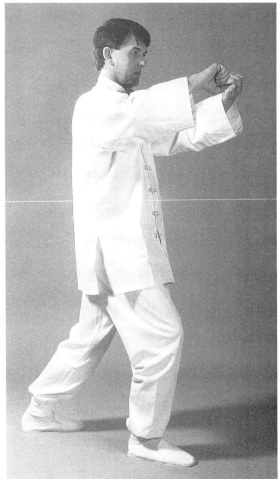

Fig. 118

2 Right foot drops slowly on to floor at a point slightly to the right and in front of left foot, while weight is shifted on to right leg to form a bow step. At the same time, drop both hands and gradually clench the fists. Then the hands make an arc upward and forward from the sides to the front, coming face to face at ear level in a pincer movement, knuckles facing obliquely upward. Distance between fists is about 10–20 cm. Look at right fist. (Figs. 117–118)

Points to remember: Hold head and neck erect. Keep waist and hips relaxed and fists loosely clenched. Keep shoulders low and allow elbows to fall naturally with arms slightly bent. Face 10 o'clock in the final position.

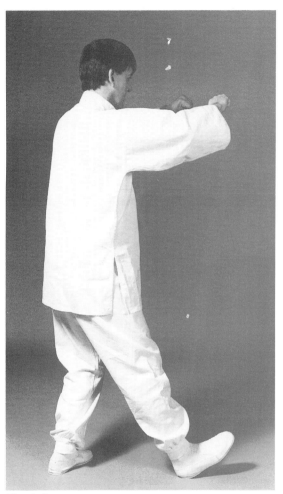

Fig. 119

Fig. 120

SERIES V

Form 15   Turn and Kick with Left Heel

1   Bend left leg and sit back. Turn body to the left (6 o'clock) with toes of right foot pointing inward. Simultaneously, open fists and separate hands in a circular movement and extend them sideways a little above shoulder level, palms facing forward. Look at left hand. (Figs. 119–120)

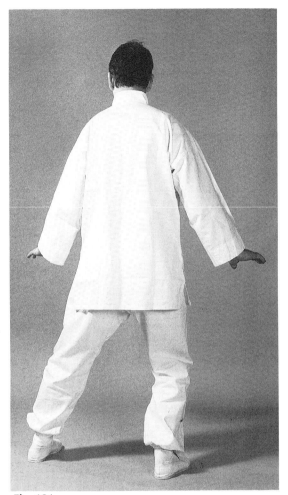

Fig. 121

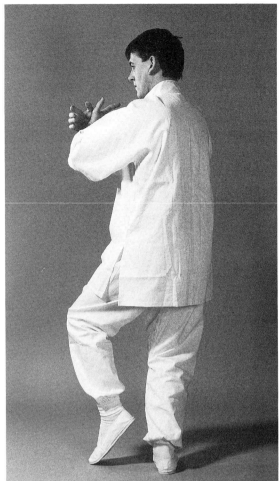

Fig. 122

2   Weight is shifted on to right leg. Bring left foot to the side of the right and rest its toes on floor. At the same time, circle both hands downward and to the sides and then inward and to the front until they cross in front of chest, with the back of right hand against the inside of left wrist, both palms facing inward. Look forward to the left. (Figs. 121–122)

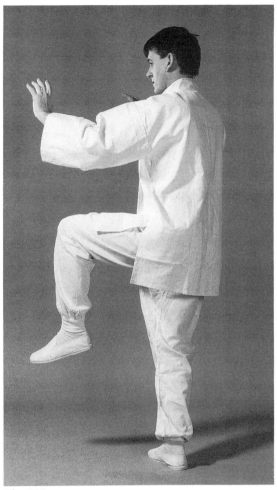

Fig. 123

Fig. 124

3 Separate hands and extend them sideways at shoulder level, elbows slightly bent and palms facing outward. Meanwhile, raise left leg with bent knee and then thrust foot gradually forward towards 4 o'clock. Look at left hand. (Figs. 123–124)

Points to remember: The same as those for Form 13, except that 'right' and 'left' are reversed. Face 4 o'clock in the final position.

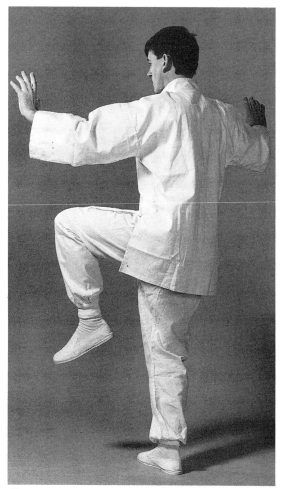

Fig. 125

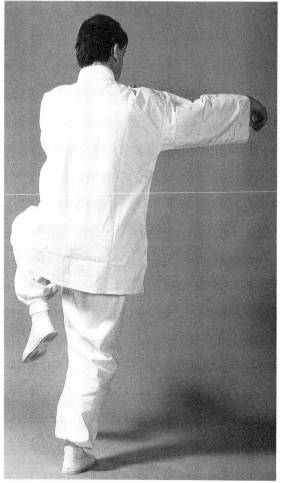

Fig. 126

SERIES VI

Form 16   Push Down and Stand on One Leg – Left Style

1   Pull back left foot and keep it suspended by bending knee so that thigh is level. Turn torso to the right (7 o'clock). Form a right hooked hand, while left palm is turned up and makes an arc upward to the right side until it comes in front of right shoulder and faces obliquely inward. Look at right hand. (Figs. 125–126)

2   Crouch slowly on right leg, stretching left leg sideways towards 2–3 o'clock. Left hand is extended sideways along the inner side of left leg, palm facing forward. Look at left hand. (Figs. 127–128)

Points to remember: When right leg is bent in a full crouch, turn toes of right foot slightly outward and straighten left leg with toes turned slightly inward; both soles are flat on floor. Keep toes of left foot in line with heel of right foot. Do not lean upper part of body too far forward.

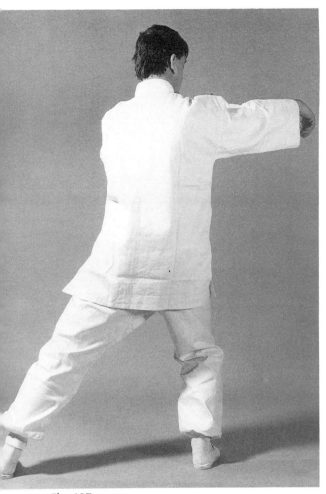

Fig. 127

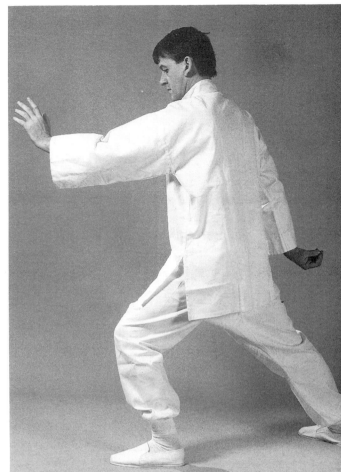

Fig. 129

3 Using heel as pivot, turn toes of left foot slightly outward so that they come in line with the outstretched leg; turn toes of right foot inward while right leg straightens and left leg bends. Weight is thus being shifted on to left leg. Torso turns slightly to the left (4 o'clock) and then rises slowly in a forward movement. At the same time, left arm continues to extend forward, with palm facing the right side, while right hand drops behind the back, with bunched fingertips pointing backward. Look at left hand. (Fig. 129)

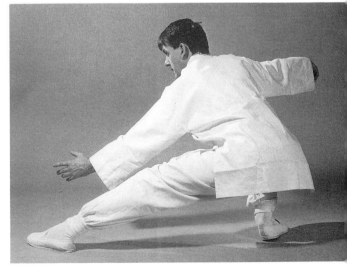

Fig. 128

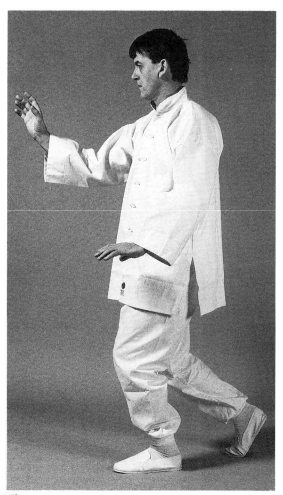

Fig. 130

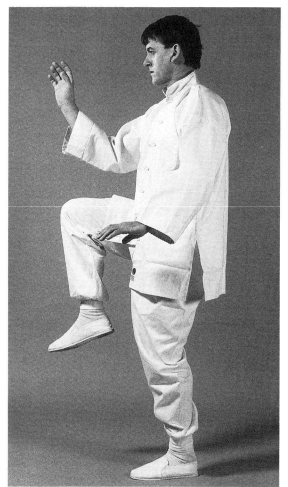

Fig. 131

4 Raise right foot gradually and bend right knee so that thigh is level. At the same time, open right hand and swing it past the outer side of right leg and then upward to the front, until the bent elbow is just above right knee, fingers pointing up and palm facing the left side. Lower left hand to the side of left hip, palm facing downward. Look at right hand. (Figs. 130–131)

Points to remember: Keep torso upright. Bend the standing leg slightly. Toes should point naturally downward as right foot is raised. Face 3 o'clock in the final position.

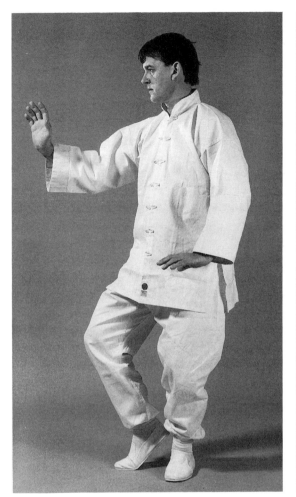

Fig. 132

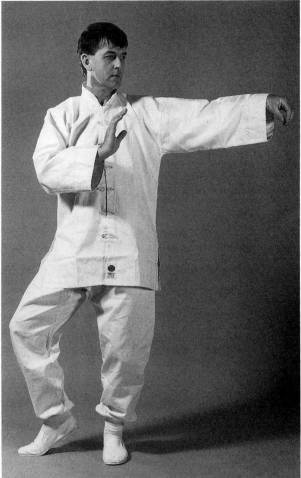

Fig. 133

SERIES VI

Form 17   Push Down and Stand on One Leg – Right Style

1   Put right foot down in front of the left and rest its toes on floor. Turn body to the left (12 o'clock), using left toes as a pivot. At the same time, left hand is raised sideways and upward to shoulder level and is turned into a hooked hand, while right hand, following body turn, moves in an arc until it comes in front of left shoulder with fingers pointing up. Look at left hand. (Figs. 132–133)

93

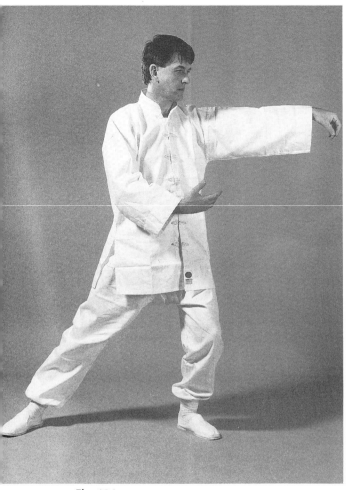

Fig. 134

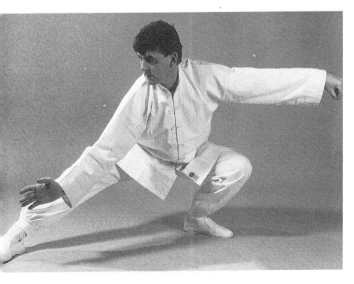

Fig. 135

Fig. 136

2   Repeat movements in 2 of Form 16, reversing 'right' and 'left.' (Figs. 134–135)

3   Repeat movements in 3 of Form 16, reversing 'right' and 'left.' (Fig. 136)

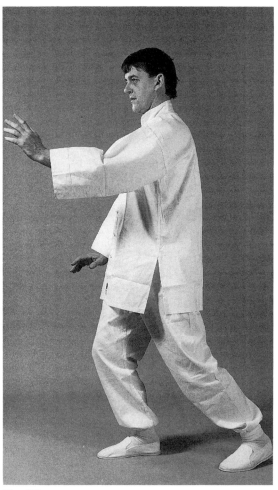

Fig. 137

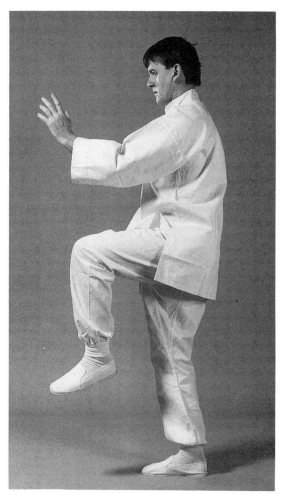

Fig. 138

4 Repeat movements in 4 of Form 16, reversing 'right' and 'left.' (Figs. 137–138)

Points to remember: Raise right foot slightly before crouching and stretching right leg sideways. Other points are the same as those for Form 16, except that 'right' and 'left' are reversed. Face 3 o'clock in the final position.

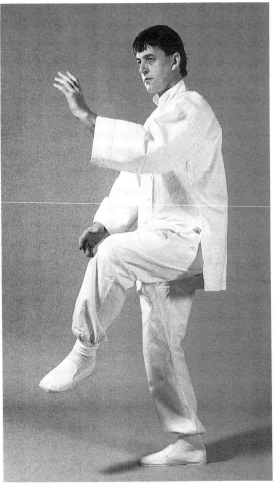

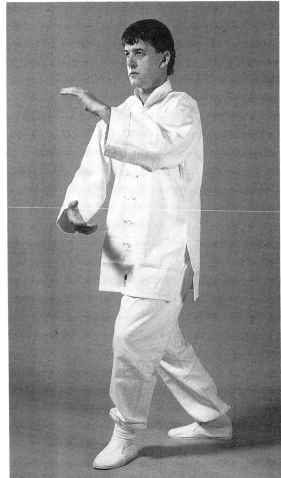

Fig. 139

Fig. 140

SERIES VII

Form 18 Work at Shuttles on Both Sides

1 Turn body to the left (1 o'clock). Left foot drops on floor in front of right foot, with toes pointing outward. With right heel slightly raised, bend both knees to form a half 'seat on crossed legs.' At the same time, make a hold-ball gesture before left part of chest, left hand on top. Then move right foot to the side of left foot and rest its toes on floor. Look at left forearm. (Figs. 139–141)

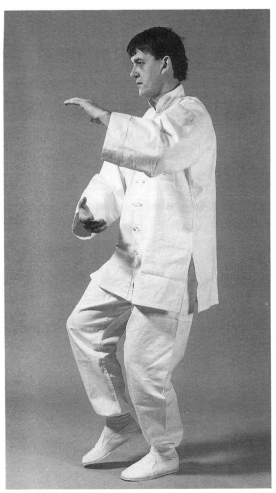

Fig. 141

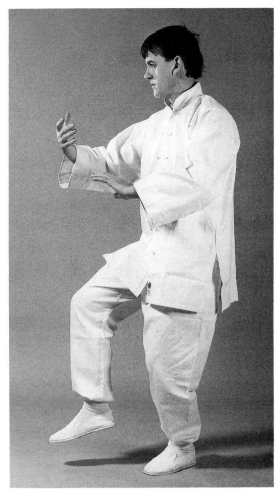

Fig. 142

2 Body turns to the right (4 o'clock) and right foot takes a step forward towards 4–5 o'clock to form a bow step. At the same time, right hand moves upward, stopping just above right temple with palm turned obliquely upward. Left hand first moves downward to the left side and then pushes forward and upward to nose level, with palm facing forward. Look at left hand. (Figs. 142–144)

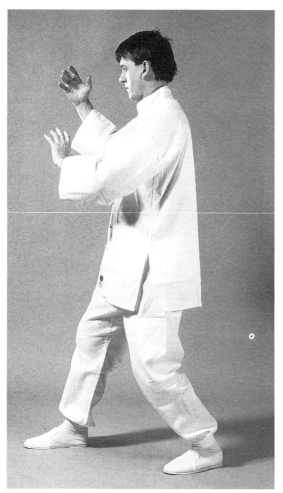

Fig. 143

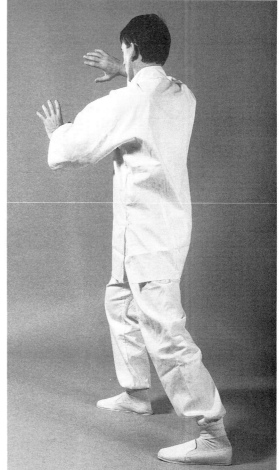

Fig. 144

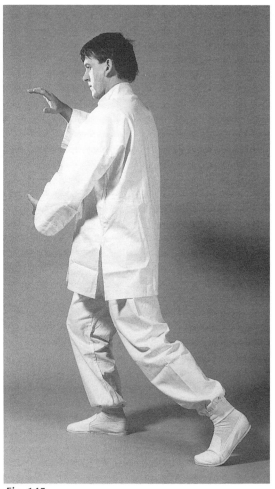

Fig. 145

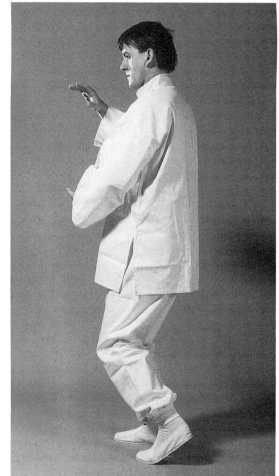

Fig. 146

3 Turn body slightly to the right (5 o'clock), shifting weight slightly backward, with toes of right foot turned outward a bit. Then weight is shifted back on to right leg. Place left foot by the side of right foot with toes on floor. Meanwhile, make a hold-ball gesture in front of right part of chest, right hand on top. Look at right forearm. (Figs. 145–146)

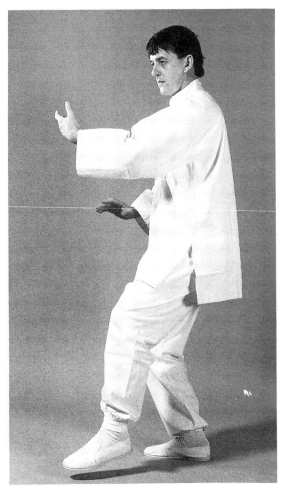

Fig. 147

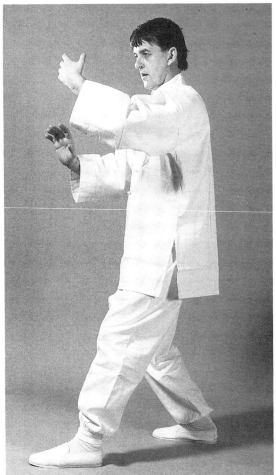

Fig. 148

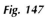

4 Repeat movements in 2, reversing 'right' and 'left.' (Figs. 147–149)

Points to remember: Do not not lean forward when pushing hands forward, or shrug shoulders when raising hands. Movements of hands should be coordinated with those of waist and legs. Transverse distance between heels in bow step is about 30 cm. Face 2 o'clock in the final position.

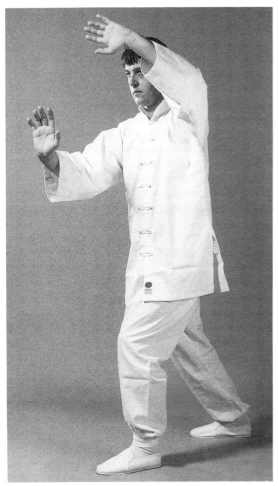

Fig. 149

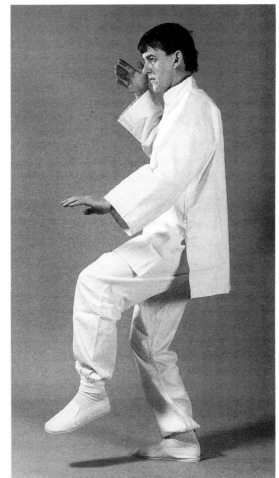

Fig. 150

SERIES VII

Form 19   Needle at Sea Bottom

1 Right foot takes half a step forward. Weight is shifted on to right leg as left foot moves forward a bit with toes coming down on floor to form a left empty step. At the same time, turn body slightly to the right (3–4 o'clock). Lower right hand in front of body, then raise it up to the side of right ear and, with body turning towards 2–3 o'clock, thrust it obliquely downward in front of body, with palm facing to the left and fingers pointing obliquely downward. Simultaneously, left

101

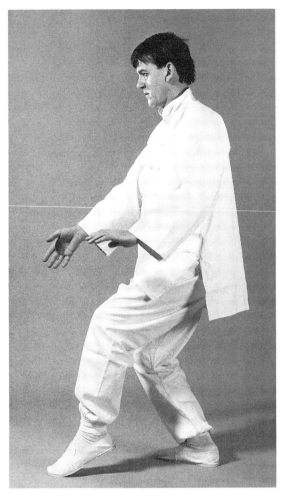

Fig. 151

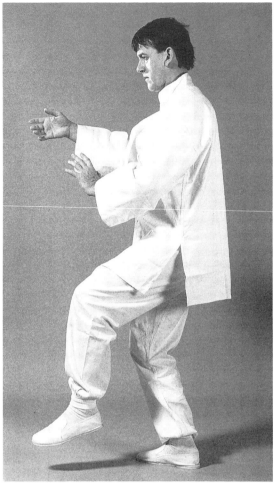

Fig. 152

hand makes an arc forward and downward to the side of left hip with palm facing downward and fingers pointing forward. Look at floor ahead. (Figs. 150–151)

Points to remember: Turn body first slightly to the right and then to the left. Do not lean too far forward. Keep head erect and buttocks in. Left leg is slightly bent. Face 3 o'clock in the final position.

SERIES VII

Form 20   Flash the Arm

Turn body slightly to the right (4 o'clock). Left foot takes a step forward to form a bow step. At the same time, raise right arm with elbow bent until the hand stops just above right temple. Turn palm obliquely upward with thumb pointing downward. Raise left hand slightly and push it forward at nose level with palm facing forward. Look at left hand. (Figs. 152–154)

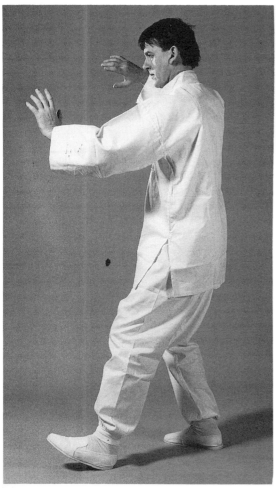

Fig. 153

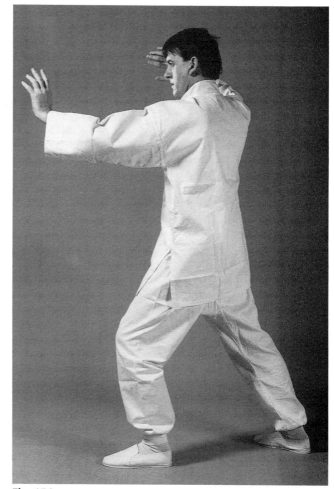

Fig. 154

Points to remember: Hold torso in an erect and natural position. Relax waist and hips. Do not straighten left arm. Keep muscles of the back relaxed. In pushing palm forward, the movement should be in harmony with that of taking the bow step. Transverse distance between heels should not exceed 10 cm. Face 3 o'clock in the final position.

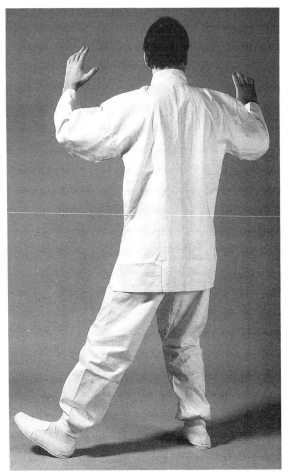

Fig. 155

SERIES VIII

Form 21   Turn, Deflect Downward, Parry and Punch

1 Sit back and shift weight on to right leg. Body turns to the right (6 o'clock), with toes of left foot turned inward. Then shift weight again on to left leg. Simultaneously with body turn, right hand circles towards the right and downward and then, with fingers clenched into a fist, moves past abdomen to the side of left ribs with knuckles up. At the same time, raise left arm above head with palm turned obliquely upward. Look forward. (Figs. 155–156)

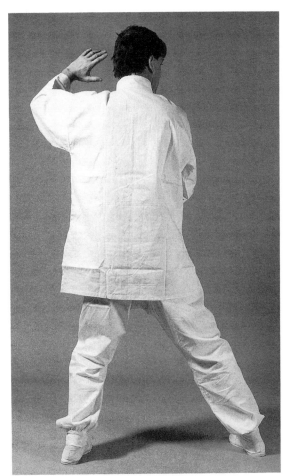

Fig. 156A

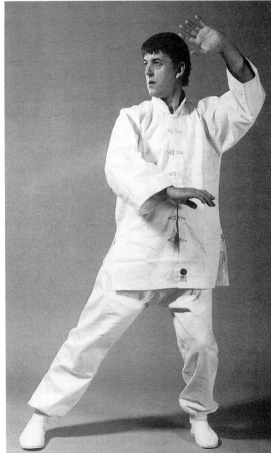

Fig. 156B

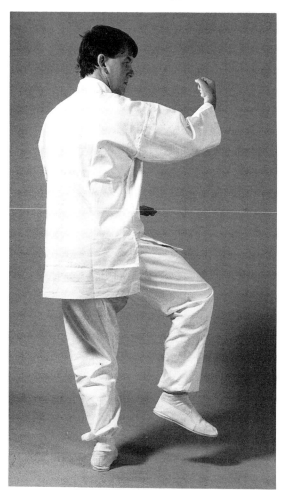

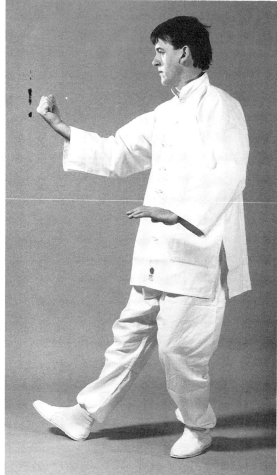

Fig. 157A

Fig. 157B

2 Turn body to the right (8 o'clock). Right fist thrusts upward and forward in front of chest with knuckles turned down. Left hand lowers to the side of left hip with palm turned downward and fingers pointing forward. At the same time, draw back right foot and, without stopping or allowing it to touch floor, take a step forward with toes turned outward. Look at right fist. (Figs. 157–158)

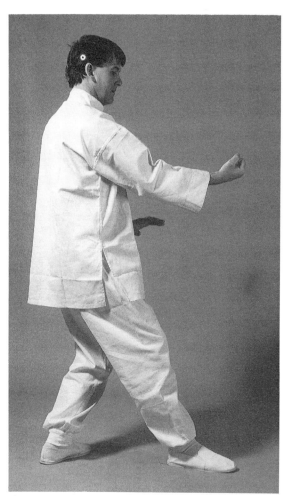

Fig. 158

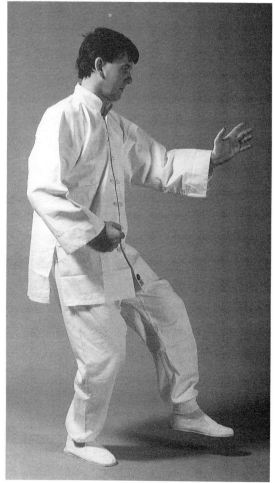

Fig. 159

3 Weight is shifted on to right leg and left foot takes a step forward. Meanwhile, parry with left hand moving up and forward from the left side in a circular movement, palm turned slightly downward, and pull right fist in a curve back to the side of right waist with knuckles turned downward. Look at left hand. (Figs. 159–160)

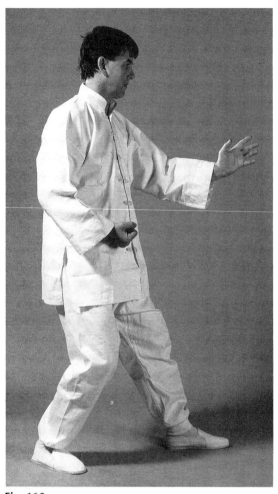

Fig. 160

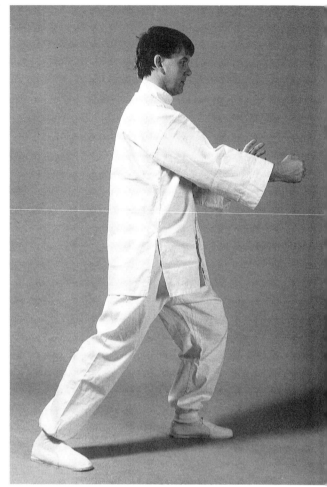

Fig. 161

4 Left leg bends to form a bow step. Meanwhile, right fist strikes forward at chest level with the back of hand facing the right side. Pull left hand back to the side of right forearm. Look at right fist. (Fig. 161)

Points to remember: Clench right fist loosely. While pulling back the fist, forearm is first turned inward and then outward. While the fist strikes forward, right shoulder follows the movement and extends a bit forward. Hold shoulder and elbows down. Face 9 o'clock in the final position.

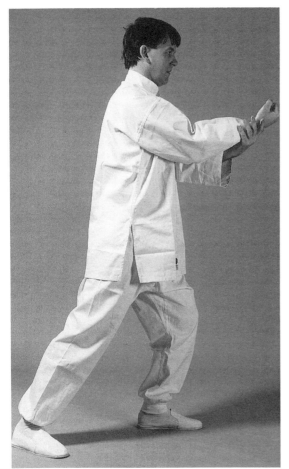

Fig. 162

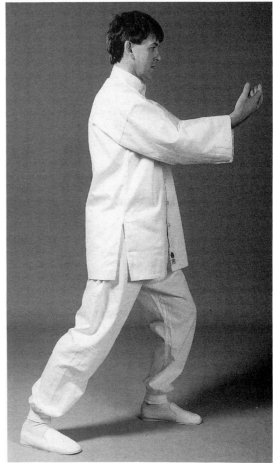

Fig. 163

SERIES VIII

Form 22   Apparent Close-up

1 Left hand stretches forward from below right wrist; right fist opens. Turn palms up, separate hands and pull them back slowly. Sit back with toes of left foot raised, shifting weight on to right leg. Look forward. (Figs. 162–164)

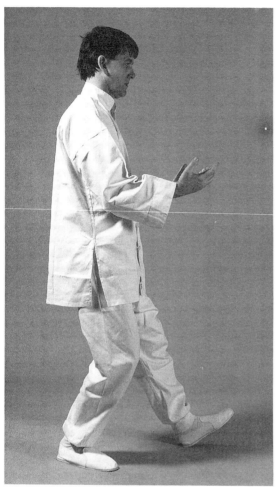

Fig. 164

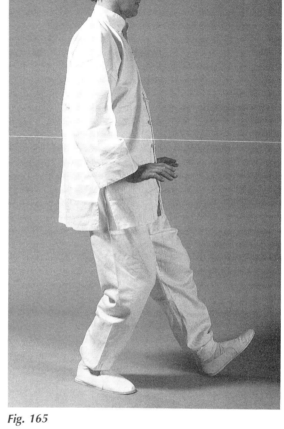

Fig. 165

2 Turning palms down in front of chest, push them downward past abdomen and then forward and upward. The movement finishes with wrists at shoulder level, palms facing forward. At the same time, bend left leg to form a bow step. Look between the hands. (Figs. 165–167)

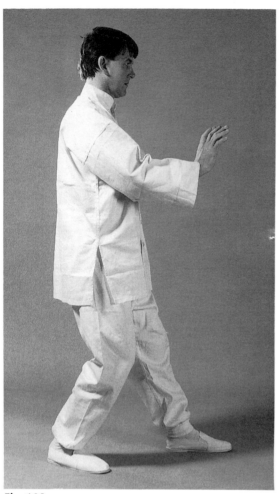

Fig. 166

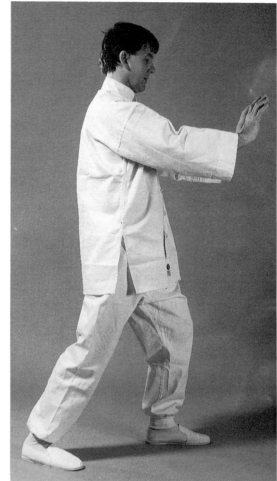

Fig. 167

Points to remember: Do not lean backward when sitting back. Keep buttocks in. Relax shoulders and turn elbows a bit outward as arms are pulled back in unison with body movement. Do not pull arms back straight. The extended hands should be no farther than shoulder-width apart. Face 9 o'clock in the final position.

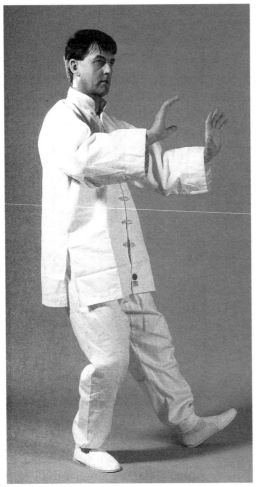

Fig. 168

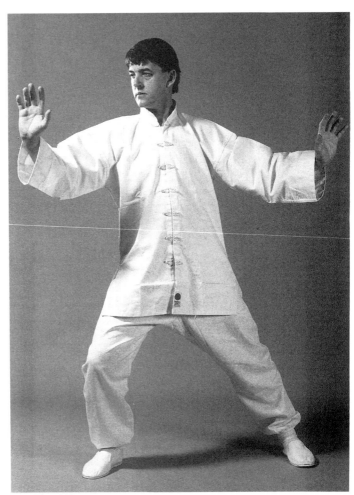

Fig. 169

SERIES VIII

Form 23   Cross Hands

1 Bend right knee and sit back, shifting weight on to right leg. Body turns to the right (1 o'clock) as toes of left foot turn inward. Following body turn both hands move to the sides in a circular movement at shoulder level, with palms facing forward and elbows slightly bent. Meanwhile, toes of right foot turn slightly outward and weight is shifted on to right leg to form a side bow step. Look at right hand. (Figs. 168–169)

2 Weight is slowly shifted on to left leg and toes of right foot turn inward. Then bring right foot towards the left so that they are parallel and shoulder-width apart; legs are gradually straightened. At the same time, move both hands down and cross them in front of abdomen, then raise the crossed hands to chest level with wrists at shoulder level, right hand on the outside and palms facing inward. Look straight forward. (Figs. 170–171)

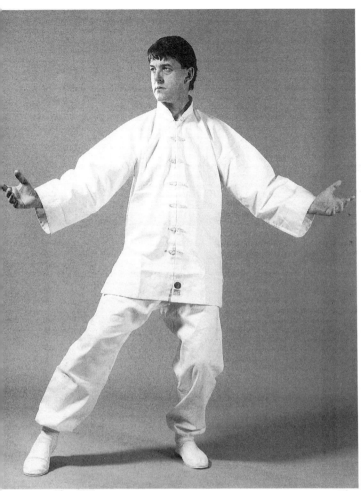

Fig. 170

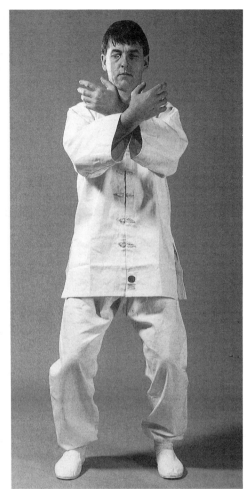

Fig. 171

Points to remember: Do not lean forward when separating or crossing hands. When taking the parallel stance, keep body naturally erect, with head held straight and chin tucked slightly inward. Keep arms rounded in a comfortable position, with shoulders and elbows held down. Face 12 o'clock in the final position.

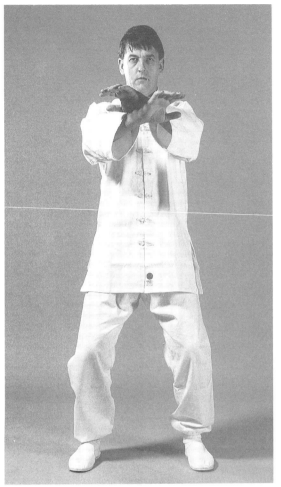

Fig. 172

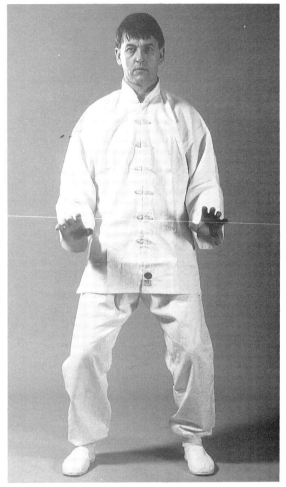

Fig. 173

SERIES VIII

Form 24   Closing Form

Turn palms forward and downward while lowering both hands gradually to the side of hips. Look straight forward. (Figs. 172–174)

Points to remember: Keep whole body relaxed and slowly draw a deep breath (exhalation to be somewhat prolonged) as hands are lowered. Bring left foot to the side of right foot after your breath is even. Take a walk for complete recovery.

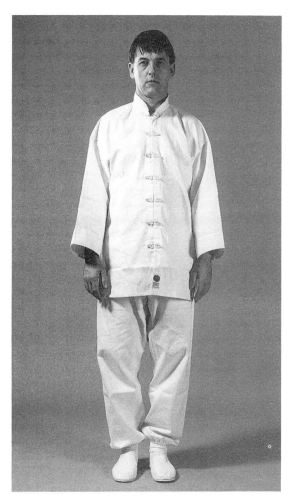

Fig. 174

6 Pushing Hands (Tuishou)

Pushing hands is the two-person exercise customarily taught after one has finished learning the tai-chi solo form. It is sometimes explained as the intermediary stage between practice of the solo form for health and the application of its movements in self-defence.

The Four Sides

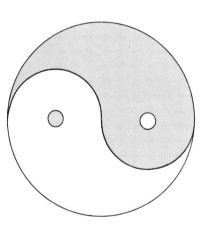

Pushing hands illustrates perfectly the meaning behind the tai-chi philosophy of the Great Polarity and its union of negative and positive forces (Yin and Yang). Its motion essentially follows an endless circular figure of eight, which calls to mind the tai-chi diagram (see left).

(1) A raises his arms (*peng*); (2) which B pulls (*lyu*); (3) A squeezes his arms (*ji*); (4) which B presses (*an*). A and B then switch actions. With practice, the movements become so smooth it is hard to say at which point one begins and another ends. The arms remain in contact and the feet remain fixed to the ground, at the basic stage.

These four actions are known as the 'four sides', and are described in the relevant section of the tai-chi classic. They are the foundation of the pushing hands exercise and the core of the theory of endless motion, which is the hallmark of tai-chi.

What is their origin and meaning?

These four actions, which constitute the core of the application of the Great Polarity Theory to the practice of tai-chi boxing, are directly attested by the Chen family records, though these do not mention the word tai-chi or its philosophy. Here is the Chen family version:

> Raise, Pull, Squeeze, Press must be in earnest.
> Up and down in succession, men find it hard to advance.
> Let him, with giant force, come to strike me:
> See how four ounces deflects a thousand pounds!
> Draw him on to fall into the void, join and then expel.
> Stick, Adhere, Commit and Follow.
> Don't drop or go against.

This is simple and direct. The basic ideas of the Great Polarity Boxing Theory (see Chapter 4) are here in a nutshell; self-defence, neutralization of superior force and even the phrase 'four ounces deflects a thousand pounds'. In motion divided, 'in stillness joined', appears to be the philosophical rendering of 'join and then expel'.

So which came first, the boxing or the philosophy? The boxer or the philosopher? Graduates from the school of hard knocks would seem more likely candidates for the ivory tower of philosophers than the reverse. Finally the two schools merged.

How then did boxing evolve into something involving actions like Raise, Pull, Squeeze, Press? There is little hint of them in Qi Jiquang's *Boxing Classic*, nor of the underlying concept of 'sticking' (adhering), which is described in the *Great Polarity Boxing Theory*.

Yet 'sticking' is a concept that can be found in Qi Jiquang's spear-fighting drills. The Chen family tradition and records include a two-man spear-sticking routine which has four basic movements (*sa-quang daizha fa*). Each movement involves a defensive drawing-out of the attack. It is easy to see how this basic fencing technique of maintaining contact with the opponent's blade or spear pole could have .evolved, for a weapon having been dispensed with, into the pushing hands exercise we know today.

There is support for this hypothesis in the tradition that Yang Lu-chan became known as Peerless Yang (Yang Wudi) for his skill with the spear, with which he could uproot an opponent. (Uproot is the term used to describe the unbalancing of an opponent, sometimes lifting him off the floor. Great masters were reckoned to be of such high skill that their opponents would literally fly through the air.)

The 'Negative Talisman Spear' axioms, ascribed to a 'Mr Wang of Shanji' and dated 1795, include the phrase 'Stick and Follow, don't let go'. Tang Hao discovered this manuscript, which includes a copy of the *Tai-chi Boxing Classic*, in a Peking market.

The practice of pushing hands is by no means confined to tai-chi in China, or to the 'soft' martial arts styles. For example: wingchun boxing, which developed in Guangong and Hong Kong, has a method of 'sticky hands' (*chisau*). White Crane Boxing, developed in Fujian and Taiwan, has a hard 'sticking hands' exercise. This employs a 'swallowing and spitting-out' (Mandarin: *tuntu*) technique, which is the same in principle as the Chen family 'join and then expel'.

What kind of benefits can be derived from pushing hands?

This is the key which the *Great Polarity Boxing Theory* calls

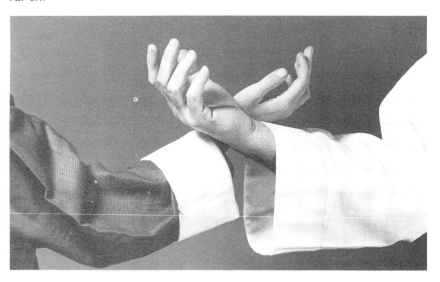

Engaging arms sensitivity drill: single-handed push practice

'understanding power' (*dhong jing*). It has the added advantage, compared to solo practice, that one has a partner to work with. The object is to learn to follow and turn an opponent's force. It is a good way to relax and unwind, looking for areas of undetected tension. It is an efficient means of correcting errors in posture and double weighting.

As the correct posture is found and movements begin to flow from the waist, deep abdominal breathing is automatically promoted. Hence it is desirable to practise in the fresh air.

After mastery of basic pushing hands, one can go at a higher stage to learn *da lyu* (the 'four corners'), which involves stepping forwards, backwards and sideways. Then there is the 'free hand' (*sanshou*) set of fixed sparring with forty-four paired attacks and counters including punches, chops and kicks.

These two-man/woman exercises add an element of stimulating competition and, if done with proper attention and control, greatly enhance the pleasure and interest of the solo practice.

Circular versus Straight, Hard versus Soft, Slow versus Fast

There has been a tendency among certain schools, particularly the dominant Yang school and students of the late Cheng Man-ching, to emphasize softness even more vigorously than has Lao Tzu, the founder of Taoism himself.

This is not in accord with the philosophy either of the tai-chi theory or the *Change Classic* from which it ultimately derives. This philosophy stems from the concept of hard and soft in their proper place. As the tai-chi *Great Polarity Boxing Theory* puts it: 'Negative does not leave positive. Positive does not leave negative.'

As a step in teaching beginners, particularly the old or weak, it is well to begin with softness. Yet for those who desire a greater degree of exertion, the vigorous may also be taught. Chen family tai-chi shows that tai-chi is by no means limited to soft, slow and circular motions. Movements may be speeded up. As the *Theory* says: 'Move fast and the reaction is fast'.

The movement is based on the circle, but it is not limited to the circle. In the solo exercise, as in the two-person forms, there is both a storing-up and letting-go. This is only hinted at in the *Theory*: Following contraction, proceed to extend. In the 'Mental Understanding' (see Chapter 7), it is made perfectly plain:

> 'Store power as if drawing a bow.
> Shoot forth power as if loosing an arrow.'

Sport, Health and Self-defence

There is a tendency among schools to belittle others. This is hinted at in the tai-chi *Theory*: 'This skill has many side schools . . .' In the seventeenth century, Huang Lizhou's claimed the supposedly Taoist Internal School (Neijia), to be far superior to Buddhist shaolin boxing.

Nowadays, tai-chi teachers proclaim the virtues of the 'soft' tai-chi over the 'hard' karate or shaolin. It should be remembered there is a hardness of the mind (and heart), as well as of the body. They don't necessarily go together! At one extreme, some tai-chi teachers have been known to condemn virtually all other forms of physical exercise, including running, as harmful to the *qi* (breath).

In the present writer's experience (based on twenty years of tai-chi practice and observation), tai-chi is an excellent conditioner for all sports. Running, weightlifting (in moderation), shaolin boxing, yoga, callisthenics, push-ups and stretching are all excellent forms of exercise and are, in fact, complements to advanced tai-chi. The development of good muscle tone and flexibility are self-promoting and not mutually opposed.

In order to derive full benefit from tai-chi, the fallacy of exclusivity must be overcome.

'Uprooting' and Competitive Pushing Hands

Lightness is the key. As the 'Mental Understanding' theory says, 'The whole body must be light and sensitive.' This does not mean soft and floppy.

One partner must make some attack or put up some resistance in order to test the other – just as one cannot play a football match without a ball.

The concept of fencing is helpful. One should work to fend off blows by sticking and adhering to the opponent. Then if one breaks his balance he may be uprooted.

The object is not simply to hoist the opponent into the air, as seen sometimes at demonstrations. When this is achieved, it usually involves some form of joint lock (usually of the elbows), self-induced or otherwise. It can look spectacular, even magical, but it is not a technique of invincible self-defence. Nor is the object to stand immovable against a push. This 'rooting', like its opposite 'uprooting' is a technique that may be practised to strengthen the legs and posture, but it is no substitute for mobility, the 'running' of the tai-chi *Theory*.

On no account should pushing hands be allowed to generate into a tug-of-war or 'fighting bulls' (*dou niu*) in the manner of a sumo wrestler, but without the proper outfit.

One important point, whose neglect frequently leads to the above type of misapplication, is the use of wrist or arm as the point of contact in sticking, rather than the palms of the hands. Use of the hands in contact with an opponent denies one the possibility of striking (lightly, in practice!) with them. At the same time over-concentration on the hands and the innate tendency to grab will slow down one's movement, making it impossible to control the opponent, or use the power of one's waist.

To achieve a high level in this aspect of tai-chi study, it is absolutely necessary to have a teacher and someone to practise with. Although many people only have a minor interest in these exercises for self-defence, they will find that they can still develop their skill at softness and suppleness to a higher degree.

Two-person Drill

Tai-chi pushing hands may be termed the sparring method of the system, and is so designed that practice may locate undetected stiffness in technique. In China nowadays there are national and international contests whereby both contestants practise competitive pushing within a fixed area and attempt to push out the other. I have not heard favourable comments regarding this modernization and some cognoscenti feel this 'hard' element could take it along the path of competitive judo.

Pushing-hand practice nonetheless is an excellent and stimulating exercise using the whole body and responds to the energy of your partner. It is generally studied after mastery of the solo exercise has been delivered and gives stimulation to practice. Many purists consider that the root of the tai-chi exercise is the section under 'grasp sparrows tail', which are the same move-

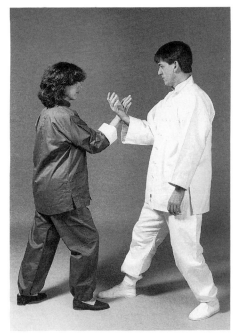

Fig. 1

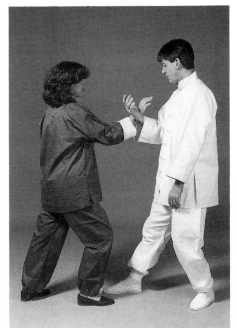

Fig. 2

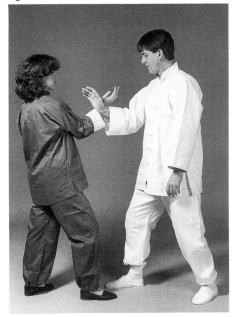

Fig. 3

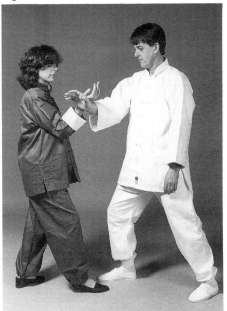

Fig. 4

1. *A and B stand facing each other. A pushes forward with right palm; B turns the waist and rests weight on the back leg*
2. *B, having neutralized A's push, begins to push back*
3. *A transfers the weight to the back leg and turns the waist to neutralize the push*
4. *The cycle is then completed as B pushes forward and A prepares to continue the sequence*

121

ments performed in the pushing hands practice.

The series of photos are two simple sensitivity drills that allow two people to practise the principles of tai-chi in a moving and joining fashion.

In the first drill both partners stand facing each other with the same hand and leg forward, arms crossing at the wrist. One party instigates a gentle push to the chest of the other, this is deflected by the other transfering their weight to the back leg, turning the waist and neutralizing the push by keeping the hand in line with the body. You will come to a point where to continue the movement would mean disengagement and overbalance. Instead, the person who has 'warded off' then changes and begins to push, transferring the weight to the forward foot, at the same time turning the waist and creating a smooth change from one movement to the next. As the practice continues, the movement itself takes over and it is possible to become more aware of your balance and the energy being put out by your partner. Do not use arm strength but allow the arm to express the energy generated by the waist and legs.

The second drill consists of each person performing the same movements facing each other. The two movements are 'brush knee hip twist' and 'ward off', interwoven in a continuous movement. First make sure you are both standing with the same foot forward. Stand close enough so that the arms can interconnect whilst keeping the shoulders relaxed. During this exercise the body changes the weight from the front leg to the back in a smooth action, whilst co-ordinating the hands and waist in a smooth continuous performance of the techniques.

The purpose of this exercise is to educate the body to become aware of sensitivity. Awareness of your partner's movement is clearer if you extend your energy forward a fraction. This allows you to read their intention and direction of energy.

Don't overreach. Maintain your balance throughout the sequence, allowing the arms to flow smoothly around your partners'. Causing both hands to move simultaneously whilst performing with a partner adds an interesting dimension to the practice. Following the photos step-by-step you will soon experience a flow of energy being exchanged. Adhering gently to your partner's movement allows you to follow the principles of tai-chi movement.

First, one partner makes a 'brush knee hip twist', which is neutralized by 'ward off', which then changes back into 'brush knee hip twist' and so on. Practising with the eyes closed is the next step which allows you to become more aware of your sensory responses.

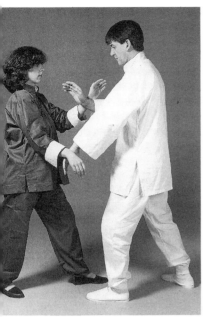
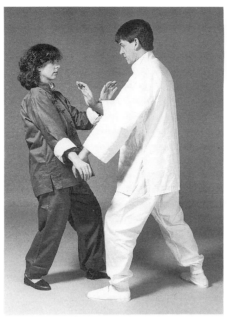
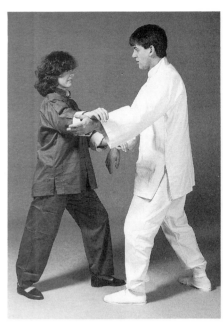

Fig. 1   **Fig. 2**   **Fig. 3**

1. Partners engage arms as shown, B with both arms inside A's
2. A leans on back leg and turns waist slightly to ward off B's push to the centre
3. A circles both hands until both are inside B's hands
4. A begins the adopt the brush knee hip twist posture as B prepares to ward off
5. B wards off to the right. A is careful not to overreach
6. B then circles the arms in the prescribed manner and begins to brush knee hip twist. A prepares to ward off to the right   7.   Thus the cycle starts again

Fig. 4   **Fig. 5**   **Fig. 6**

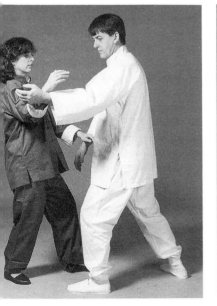
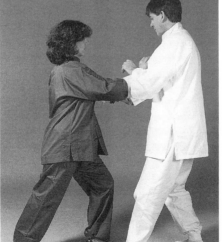
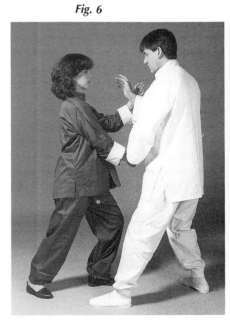

Along with the solo form I taught this sensitivity drill to the cast of 'Real Dreams' by Trevor Griffiths, both in Massachusetts (USA) and the Royal Shakespeare Company, London. The cast had to perform tai-chi in the play and had thirty days in which to learn. All actors suffer performance nerves, and both casts practised the sensitivity drill before performance and claimed that it allowed them to centre themselves as well as balance their energy and calm themselves before the curtain came up.

The drill is useful because there is no 'competition' and allows you to follow your partner and they you. A living example of this in practice are the ice skating champions, Torvill and Dean, who in their performances always exhibited a tactile grace that I have only previously witnessed in the performances of tai-chi masters.

In teaching this drill I have generally found that men have greater difficulty in the early stages because of their psychological investment in arm strength. In fact, the gentler your partner, the more you have to relax. Sometimes a couple may request me to referee their attempts to relax, accusing their partners of stiffness. This is often due to stiffness in the wrist in not allowing the arms to fold around each other as one movement is changing into the other. The exercise balances the energy between your two arms and creates the awareness of one movement flowing into the other in a smooth flowing action.

Standing with the left foot forward would mean your left hand moving in a clockwise direction and the right hand in an anticlockwise direction. My teacher Zhang Yizhong claimed this exercise was taught to his teacher Wang Shujin by Chen-Pan-Ling, who was the leader of the martial arts community in Taiwan. It was explained that this exercise is good for the brain as it demands the involvement of the whole body, and to obtain that requires concentration of the mind.

For those who have studied tai-chi already I offer this exercise because you can teach it to someone very quickly. I find many tai-chi exponents frustrated missionaries. In the main it is more seductive to practise this with someone rather than making a few mystical passes in the air and leaving your audience confused and sometimes suspicious. Feeling is believing!

7 Mental Understanding for the Practice of the Thirteen Actions

after Wu Yuxiang (1812–80)[1]

With the mind circulate the breath,
Striving to make it sink firm.
Then it can be absorbed into the bones.

With the breath manoeuvre the body,
Striving to make it follow compliantly.
Then it can readily obey the mind.

If the spirit can be raised up,
Then there will be no danger of being slow or heavy.
This is what is meant by 'keeping the crown suspended'.

Idea and breath must be converted sensitively,
Then there is a feeling of roundness and mobility.
This is what is meant by 'inter-changing empty and full'.

In shooting forth power one must sink firm and loose clean,
Concentrating in one direction.
Stand the torso centrally erect and at ease,
Held up on eight sides.

Circulate the breath as if threading the nine-bend bead,
Leaving no cranny unreached.
Deploy power like a hundred times tempered steel,
Leaving nothing hard, unpulverized.

Its form is like a hawk seizing a rabbit,
Its spirit is like a cat catching a mouse,
In stillness it is like a mountain peak,
In motion like the Yangtze and Yellow rivers.

Tai-chi

Store power as if drawing a bow,
Shoot forth power as if loosing an arrow,
In the bent seek the straight:
Store up and then shoot forth.

Force is from the spine shot forth,
Steps are following the torso alternated.

Drawing-in is letting-loose:
Cut off and then re-connect.
To and from must have a folding action,
Advance and retreat must be interchanged.

Extremely soft and supple:
Only then extremely hard and strong.
If one can inhale and exhale:
Only then can one be sensitive and mobile.

Breath by straightness is nourished without harm.
Power by bending is stored in abundance.[2]

The mind is the commander's ensign;
The breath the flags;
The waist the banner.

First seek opening out,
Later seek tight concentration.
Then one can attain the close-knit.

First in the mind, afterwards in the body.
Abdomen relaxed, breath absorbed into the bones.
Spirit at ease, body at rest.
Constantly bear in mind and remember:

Once in motion, everything in motion;
Once at rest, everything at rest.
Tugged in motion back and forth
The breath adheres to the back
And is absorbed into the spine.

Inwardly consolidate the spirit
Outwardly show a peaceful ease.[3]
Make steps like a cat walking,
Deploy power like unwinding silk.

The whole body's concentration is in the spirit not in the breath.
If in the breath it is impeded.
He who has breath lacks force.
He who nurtures breath is pure, adamant.
Breath is like a carriage wheel,
The waist is like a carriage axle.

If he does not move,
Oneself does not move.
If he moves slightly
Oneself has moved first.

The power is as if relaxed but not relaxed,
About to open yet still unopened.
Power may be cut, the idea is not cut.

First in the mind,
Then in the body.

Once movement is commenced,
The whole body must be light and sensitive.
Above all it must be coordinated.
Let the breath be expanded freely,
The spirit inwardly absorbed.
Don't let there be deficient places,
Don't let there be protruding or caved-in places,
Don't let there be disconnected places.

Tai-chi

Its root is at the feet,
It is shot forth in the legs,
Governed in the waist,
Formed in the hands.
From feet and legs and waist
It should always be entirely one breath.
Advancing forwards, or retreating back,
One can then get the timing and get position.
If unable to get the timing or get position,
The body then becoming uncoordinated and disordered.
The fault should be sought in the waist and legs.
Upwards, downwards, forwards and backwards left and right are all thus.

All this is idea,
Not all externals.
Where there is high, there is low.
Where there is forward, there is back.
Where there is left, there is right.
Should the idea be upward,
First lodge a downward idea.

It is like, when scooping up an object, to add the idea
   of crushing it,
So that its root will be automatically broken.
Then its destruction will be speedy and without doubt.

Empty and full should be clearly distinguished:
Each place has each place's empty and full.
The whole body's every joint is in coordination,
Allowing not a hair's breadth interruption.

Long Boxing is like the Long Yangtze or the Great Sea
Surging on and on without a break.

Raise, Pull, Squeeze, Press, Grab, Cut, Elbow,
Barge – these are the Eight Trigrams.

Advance, Retreat, Look left, Turn right, Centre fixed – These are the Five Elements.

Raise, Pull, Squeeze, Press
are
The Four Sides.

Grab, Cut, Elbow, Barge
are
The Four Corners.

Advance, Retreat, Look left, Turn right, Centre fixed.
Are Metal, Wood, Water, Fire, Earth.

Together they make Thirteen Actions.

Notes

1. Translator's Note: Unlike the Theory (see Chapter 4), the *Mental Understanding* is not attributed to Wang Zongyue. It is more practical in focus and less polished in composition. Yet like the Theory, it combines quotations from various sources, including the Confucian classics, to illustrate a non-dualist philosophy of self-defence and mind-body co-ordination.
2. Mencius: 5, Gongsun chou
3. Wu-Yuek, Springs and Autumns IX: 'The way of all fighting is: inwardly consolidate the spirit, outwardly show a peaceful aspect.'

8 Meditation

According to Zen Buddhists, there are at least seven types of meditation practices which are generally employed. After each one I have written in brackets its modern application.

1. Meditation through breathing exercises – qigong, yoga
2. Meditation by concentrating one's mind on one point (qigong)
3. Meditation through visualization (art, music, literature)
4. Meditation through mantram yoga – the reciting or incantation of mystic words (transcendental meditation)
5. Meditation by absorbing one's mind in good will or devotional thoughts (religious prayer)
6. Meditation by identifying the mind essence (philosophy, psychology)
7. Meditation through movement (tai-chi, qigong, yoga, dance, running), martial arts practise

Wei-lang caused a sensation in the eighth century with his revolutionary concept of meditation, stating that it was not the art of tranquilizing the mind and that one-sided meditation is sure to lead to quietism and death. Meditation has little to do with just sitting cross-legged in contemplation, as is generally supposed by outsiders. It is about acting, moving, performing deeds, seeing, hearing, thinking, remembering – doing! – even day dreaming.

Meditation in all its forms therefore is designed to create balance within the individual, as much of the book is concerned with moving methods of meditation. The following section involves some simple techniques for static meditation that you may find useful in your overall practice.

First, let your shoulders relax . . . go on, let your shoulders relax. It's likely that they have dropped a little, but as soon as you are distracted, they will rise again. In that moment when you let your shoulders relax, you were coming to a state of meditation and your mind was not flitting from image to image, because it had come to focus on one point – that of relaxation.

Meditation for health is a continuation of that movement in

which you let your thoughts leave your mind and enter your body. This method of feeling, rather than thinking, allows the qi to flow smoothly throughout the body. This can only be achieved by relaxation. By bringing your body to a complete stop, you contain the energy within.

You should not allow your head to slump onto your chest, as this blocks the flow of energy through the neck.

When we sleep, we move unconsciously, changing our position as our bodies spontaneously adopt the most comfortable posture. In contrast, when we curl up on a couch or sit in a chair in a collapsed position, we often get up with an ache because the body weight was pressing on one point.

Drop your shoulders! Drop them! If you had to drop them again, it shows why you have to meditate to control the physical state: in the conscious state, distractions win.

Meditation is the bridge between the conscious and the unconscious and may be termed the qigong state. You will probably find, as you relax, that your breathing will deepen and the body's healing and balancing powers will begin to work. You should concentrate your mind on the breathing.

'Just a minute,' you will say. 'What about all the thoughts and ideas that emerge and bounce around my brain when I close my eyes?' Good question!

Well, sometimes I have a pen and paper handy and write down quickly things that occur to me, or that I jarringly remember. This I find releases me from continuing to think about them. Letting go, letting go, letting go is what it is all about; slowly, slowly coming to your centre. If your thoughts become too crowded, then stop. Begin to count your breath, out–in, out–in, out–in, and relax. Don't forget your face, let your face relax. With your eyes closed, you don't have to respond to the outside world.

You might feel that your face is itchy. This indicates the channels are smoothing; what you can feel is the energy flowing through your face. Don't rub or scratch, just relax and think about your breathing, which is feeding your qi.

Many people see colours, which represents the energy emanating from various organs (each has its own colour). Everybody's experience is different, unique. Everybody also possesses a talent or skill, whether or not it has been developed.

In recent times in China, with the popularity of 'qigong meditation', many individuals have shown human psychic abilities, such as telekinesis, x-ray vision and the ability to transmit 'qi' to heal and affect changes in the molecular structure of water. Whether you find these believable or not is up to you. The Chinese have set up research centres to investigate the human skills that have lain dormant in the DNA and regularly reports are finding their way into the press.

In the West, for example, some people show psychic abilities at an early age, become afraid and suppress them. The flowering of the individual comes when, through meditation, they begin to connect with themselves again. The aim is to achieve a harmony and balance of the whole person.

The biggest secret I have come across in meditation is *wu-wei*. Wu-wei is the essential ingredient that makes meditation work. What is this magical word?

Well, simply, it translates as 'nothing'. When this secret was given to me. I cracked up, I fell about on the floor, hysterical with laughter. Even now, as I write, it makes me laugh. The deepest level is nothing and the problem with nothing is that is has a name. It's interesting to note that some religions refer to God as the Nameless One, in this, I see a central point connecting many philosophies.

In the first draft of this book when the copy editor makes notes for the author there was a small question in the margin requesting an explanation of nothing, a task which philosophers throughout time have wrestled with! Leaving the remainder of the page blank might have satisfied a Zen monk, but such an earnest enquiry deserves a response.

There is an ancient Zen Koan that might be useful: 'what was your face before you were born?' Were you dead? Did you exist? Because we can accumulate knowledge of history and the mind connects and stores this information and thus we have a link through time; because we read books, watch films of events before our life started, we feel we are connected back through time. We then come to the theories regarding the beginning of the world, then the universe, until finally we come to nothing. By coming to a state of 'noneness' we leave behind the ego; by being able to lose the sense of ego we then must lose thought also, a virtually impossible task. But along the way much benefit may be derived. It's a lot like ice cream – if you never taste it you never know the flavour!

When I first began to practise meditation, I seemed to recall physically all the injuries that I had ever sustained. I felt great discomfort between the shoulder blades, a legacy of repeated punching practice. This, I found, was because my channels of energy were affected by this so-far unresolved damage to the acupuncture channels.

Acupuncture is the Chinese medical method of stimulating the channels of energy in the body to recover good health. It was not devised by the random sticking of needles into hapless victims, but came about through meditation whereby the 'qi' was felt moving around the body along channels that were mapped out and which laid the foundation for acupuncture to develop.

During meditation, when the body comes to a state of rest, you can feel energy moving throughout the body. Continued practice causes the energy to settle, and many tests have shown a change in respiration, an increase of alpha waves recorded and the practitioner enjoying improved psychological and emotional states. On reflection, doing 'nothing' is good for you!

About twenty years ago, I dislocated my shoulder and suffered much in cold weather. Practising meditation has brought much relief to this condition. My first experience was an ache and numbness that moved from my shoulder to my arm. With more practice, my forearm became numb; further practice still brought the numbness to my thumb and forefinger. This, it was explained to me, was the qi energy smoothing the channels. I no longer suffer discomfort and am convinced that if I continue to mediate I will not suffer as old age approaches.

Old age, sickness and death are the basic tenets of Buddhism. Personally, the middle one I'm willing to miss. I have to admit, though, that the groovy way to leave the planet would be in the middle of meditation: the contemplation of nothing was surely the sole mental activity before we were born and so far as I can remember, it wasn't too bad!

Society has become addicted to doing. Non-doing is an anathema to the Protestant work ethic. Yet non-doing allows us to connect with the natural elements of the universe. By coming to a stop, we become the antennae between heaven and earth. Tuning into ourselves is the ultimate journey. Many lose faith and follow -isms and trends. It comes down to how you view life . . . and its sequel!

The Five-Element Theory

Meditation can be practised both in stillness and in movement.

Spontaneous qigong, recently introduced into the West by Michael Tse, a young Chinese master, takes transcendental meditation one step further by allowing the body to move and discharge negative energy. This method helps those who find being still too difficult. Using this method, the body naturally comes to a state of balance through the movements of the five animals, which balance the qi through the collateral channels in the body. This may be termed moving meditation and is probably the quickest way to achieve health benefit in this area.

The five animals are the outward expression of the energy moving between the five internal organs which in turn relate to the five-element theory. This is best understood diagramatically:

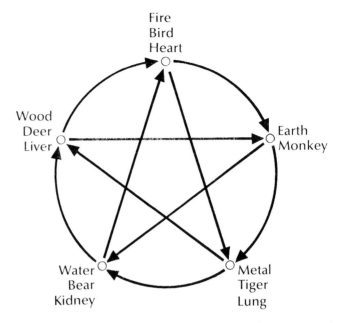

During spontaneous meditation the body adopts certain postures and gestures that have been designated animals to represent them which show the external reflecting the energy that moves internally. This cycle of creation and control smooths and balances the qi within the body.

This method should only be practised under the supervision of a qualified practitioner as some people may experience alarm and distress in the early stages of practice. This method may be learned safely after five or so sessions and the individual may then practise safely.

Meditation is now being taught in hospitals in the U K and many people seem to have benefitted. Its use as an adjunct to chemotherapy and radium treatment has shown the positive, healing aspect to meditation, which we will discuss in the next chapter.

9 How Tai-chi Improves Health and Cures Disease

In China tai-chi has long been recognized not only as a martial art but also as a health-building activity. Based on the unity of contradictions – of Yin and Yang, movement and stillness, strength and grace, emptiness and fullness etc. – its practice requires that one be naturally relaxed and still. The theory and its remarkable practical results are now attracting more and more attention.

In addition, from an exercise viewpoint, tai-chi is composed of many postures and exercises including finger movement, hand movement, wrist movement, elbow movement, arm movement, waist movement, foot movement, and eye movement.

The latest training programme set for astronauts in China, lists both tai-chi and qigong amongst the subjects of study. Seemingly, training in tai-chi and qigong can greatly increase the adaptability of astronauts, (who must endure enormous changes in their working circumstances during space flights), and thus enable scientific work to be carried out with greater efficiency.

This suggests that tai-chi has remarkable effects on human physiology and pathology and points to a rich subject for modern scientific research. This would require whole-hearted collaboration between scientists and wu-shu experts.

Tai-chi and the Soundness of the Nervous System

A master of tai-chi, Yang Chenfu, has summarized ten points in tai-chi activity:

1. Relaxing the top of the head.
2. Withdrawing the chest a little, whilst straightening the back.
3. Relaxing the waist.
4. Distinguishing between emptiness and fullness.
5. Dropping the shoulders and elbows downwards.
6. Using will rather than strength.
7. Making the upper and lower parts of the body move in harmony.
8. Coordinating the interior and the exterior.

9. Moving in a continuous way.
10. Seeking stillness in movements.

I believe from my own practice of tai-chi that the purpose of these ten points is to reach the natural state of being relaxed and still, in order to effect the natural, reciprocal transitions between Yin and Yang, emptiness and fullness, strength and grace, forward and backward movement etc. The fulfilment of these points has great significance for health, especially the soundness of the nervous system.

Confronted with an extremely complicated natural and social environment, we must call into action all our innate forces to deal with changes. This is particularly true in modern society. As competition becomes stiffer, daily life reaches a high state of tension and the cerebral nervous system reaches a corresponding state of high excitement.

Stress of this kind, over a long period, causes general weariness, decline in health and a speeding up of physiological ageing, which results in pathological changes in functions and organs. The so-called 'disease of civilization' so prevalent in today's society is mainly caused by over-intensity of the brain and over-laziness of the body.

Tai-chi, which emphasizes natural relaxation, with the stilling of both the mind and body, provides an excellent form of health care and a natural self-adjustment of the abnormalities resulting from a life of intensity and laziness.

Relaxing the body accelerates the brain into a state of being still and quiet which, in turn, helps the process of bodily relaxation. Tai-chi is performed in the body's most natural and unrestrained state. As such, it is conducive to a healthy adjustment between excitement and restraint of the central nervous system and helps to ease the nervous over-intensity of a busy life.

Furthermore, the muscle 'hunger' resulting from lack of exercise and the subsequent decline of nerve movement can be restored to normal by tai-chi practice.

A Japanese doctor pointed out in a recent medical lecture that entrepreneurs hammer their brains out in dealing with competitors and that their daily movements are dependent on cars and lifts, with very little physical activity. He is vehemently opposed to managers riding in luxury cars and strongly encourages them to stand in the tram, without taking hold of the bar. Training nerves and muscles to balance on a rocking tram is, he believes, 'a very effective way of keeping cerebral youth'. Old people lacking in exercise are most unsteady in step, slow in reactions of the senses and have difficulty keeping their balance. They are also physiologically older than they should be. By contrast, people in the same age group who have been persistent in their practice of tai-chi are mostly steady walkers, sharp in response, and their physiological ages are usually younger than their real age.

This is because tai-chi movements, being from head to limbs, with the waist as axis, bring about a series of continuous light, subtle transitions between emptiness and fullness, forward and backward movements etc. They are controlled through the coordination of feeling nerve, movement nerve and other central nerves. Because one movement is accompanied by movements of the whole body, with muscles and ligaments moving freely, tai-chi gives full exercise to the limbs and nervous system.

Intensity of work and life and accompanying over-excitement of the cerebral cortex will cause a functional imbalance of the autonomic nerve. Then, with a corresponding over-excitement of the sympathetic nerve and increasing secretion of adrenalin, the parasympathetic nerve is brought into restraint accordingly.

The functions of these two types of nerve are not in harmony. Disharmony will directly affect the autonomic-controlled movements of the internal organs, causing harm to both mind and body by quickening the heartbeat, raising the blood pressure, slowing down movements of the intestines and stomach, reducing digestive secretions and increasing the alienation of the metabolism, decreasing its assimilation.

Over a long period of time, these effects will erode one's energy, have a negative influence on the physique, and cause functional disorders of the internal organs. Tai-chi, with its relaxing, still, natural, soft and continuous movements of the body, provides an excellent way of correcting this inharmonious state.

Human beings are emotional, but being too passionate is harmful to health. Chinese medical theory lays great stress upon the negative influence of seven emotions on human beings. It believes joy, anger, melancholy, brooding, sorrow, fear and shock to be the internal factors causing disease. *Huang Di Nei Jing*, (Classics of the Yellow Emperor) at its very beginning explicitly points out that 'stillness and quietude is followed by True Qi; consolidation of spirit within drives away disease'. This book is the ancient treatise on health revered by the Chinese throughout time.

Traditional Chinese medical theory takes 'true qi' as the most essential element in life's activities. Only in a state of being quiet and still can one hope to consolidate the spirit and prevent true qi from being interrupted in its natural circulation around the body. Such a state can ensure good vigour, a fullness of positive qi and prevent susceptibility to disease.

Tai-chi sets great store by being naturally quiet and still. It demands in its practice just exactly what is good for the health. It requires one to be carefree and to forget the world and oneself in its continuous coordinated movements, involving both movement and stillness, emptiness and fullness. In this way, the seven emotions are excluded, outside stimuli are filtered and cleaned and the body is guided into its best mental and physiological state.

The functions of the various parts of the brain coordinate and synchronize, working smoothly together; the various internal secretions are balanced; the muscles relax whilst the mind and body are comfortable, moving naturally and freely, gradually entering the spiritual state of being pure and clear. As the spiritual nerve is the controlling centre of the body, this should certainly be of excellent effect in improving health and curing disease.

The Chinese hold the theory that energy in the body is part of a trinity of elements: sperm, qi and spirit; in the case of the female: blood, qi and spirit. These elements transmute into each other in western medical terminology. The phrase 'the patient's spirit is up' is often used to describe an improved condition.

A person well-trained in tai-chi will not only achieve the desired state of mind and body when practising, but will also, in daily life, be calm when confronting danger, systematic in solving problems, benign in temper and do things, according to objective laws, with full vigour. With the seven emotions remaining peaceful and moderate, a person is likely to adopt a broad-minded and optimistic attitude towards life, and can acquire a sound physical constitution and high spirit.

Tai-chi and the Respiratory and Circulatory Systems

Tai-chi requires abdominal breathing, which depends mainly on the rise and fall of the diaphragm to cause the thorax to open and close. Abdominal breathing is deep breathing. It has been proved by experiment that abdominal breathing sucks in more air than chest breathing. Normally when the diaphragm lowers one centimetre, air through the lungs will increase by 250–350 millilitre.

Abdominal breathing creates the conditions of breath needed for tai-chi, soft, even, thin and long. This not only makes the orderly physiological rhythm of the human body (and is thus good for health), but is also of benefit to those suffering from respiratory disease, because it will not increase the burden on the organs.

Because tai-chi breathing meets physiological demands, it can help to build up the physique, increase blood circulation in the organs and help both to prevent and to cure disease. For example: not a few T B patients, under the guidance of doctors, practised tai-chi gradually over a period of time. The result was either an improvement in health or a complete recovery from the disease.

With an increase of the volume of air taken into the lungs, the volume of oxygen in the body increases correspondingly, facilitating the metabolism and producing greater vigour. The more oxygen in the blood, the higher the function of the heart. Generally speaking, therefore, patients suffering from heart disease can practise tai-chi without (as happens with some other sports) greatly increasing the burden on the heart. My own experience of tai-chi is that it will improve the functions of the heart, improve health and cure disease.

Tai-chi, with its combination of movement and stillness, emptiness and fullness, relaxation and strength, and its coordination between interior and exterior parts, upper and lower parts, forward looking and backward glancing, brings all the muscles and bones into a harmonious and orderly action of withdrawals and extensions.

Tai-chi's twining movements require the limbs and body to make spiral movements. The rhythmic spiralling of muscles and ligaments has a very good effect on the elasticity of the blood vessels which they contain. This is beneficial both to the blood circulation and in the prevention of vascular sclerosis. Perhaps this is one reason why tai-chi has such an excellent effect on blood-pressure patients.

Abdominal breathing (i.e. using the diaphragm to expand the breath) makes the abdominal muscles more elastic by causing them to tense and relax in turn. The abdominal pressure is high and then low. Not only will this make the blood in the artery and veins within the abdominal cavity flow more smoothly but it will also be good for the blood circulation of all organs within this cavity. It thus quickens the metabolism of these organs and strengthens their functions and soundness.

Among these organs, the liver and the spleen are the blood reservoirs of the body. The tensing and relaxing movements of the diaphragm and the abdominal muscles will make the input and output of these two blood reservoirs function more smoothly. The blood in the whole body will be more active and strengthened, another factor in improving health and curing disease.

In the human body, the blood pressure in the veins is far below that of the arteries. When the blood within the vein circulates back to the heart, it is often retarded for various reasons. For instance, venous stasis in the womb can cause excessive or abnormal menstruation. The back-circulation of the blood in the veins also has to resist gravity, which is the reason why people who must stand frequently tend to suffer from varicose veins. These patients can make use of the pressure created by the rise and fall of the abdomen when practising tai-chi, to improve that venous back-circulation.

Many an old person with a weak physique has low abdominal muscle pressure and cannot summon the force to evacuate the bowels. The effort can prove particularly painful. If someone suffering from constipation of this kind can persist in practising tai-chi (paying special attention to abdominal breathing in order to reinforce the abdominal muscles), he or she will be able to raise abdominal pressure at will and so increase bowel movements. This constipation often disappears without the need of medicine.

The abdominal breathing of tai-chi can synchronize the movements of limbs and body and the rising and falling movements of the diaphragm. This gives a better play to the massage effect on the organs within the thoracic and abdominal cavities. These cavities house such organs as the heart, liver, spleen, lungs, kidney, stomach, small intestine, large intestine, gall bladder, bladder etc. – most of the important organs for life.

They are all located near the diaphragm and are massaged, directly or indirectly, by its rise and fall. This rhythmic massage helps the circulation of blood and qi within those organs, strengthening their metabolic functions, coordinating their orderly relations with each other and greatly improving their soundness.

This in turn influences the autonomic nerve and the central nervous system and is conducive to their correct functioning. Patients suffering from some inner organ diseases have improved in health or even recovered fully after a period of practising tai-chi.

Tai-chi differs from Western sports in that it emphasizes the 'inner *gongfu*'. It not only demands that the limbs be fleet and quick in reaction, but also sets great store by coordinated continuity between upper and lower parts of the body and between the interior and exterior. By combining the outward activity with the inner organ movements, it improves the soundness of the whole.

Tai-chi and Traditional Chinese Medical Theory

Tai-chi is recognized as a form of wu-shu activity, nurtured by the scientific and cultural thought of Chinese tradition. It fully embodies Chinese traditional philosophy's principle of tai-chi Yin and Yang. It is closely connected with Chinese traditional medical theory.

Traditional Chinese medical theory believes that the life activity of the body is closely linked in every aspect with the universe, the seasons and every natural thing. The organs of the body, the exterior and the interior of the main and collateral channels along which vital energy passes, the spirit and the form of the body are all considered as a related and mutually interacted whole.

That is, traditional Chinese medical theory has an all-encompassing conception of the heaven, earth, spirit and human body, and views them as an organic whole. To use a term from modern systems theory, we may describe the human body as a super-enormous system, among which every sub-system or factor is directly or indirectly associated with the others, acting upon them and affecting them.

This theory also states that qi, the most essential element or energy, forming everything (including the human body), in the universe. Qi can be divided into Yin and Yang, a unity of contradictions. The heaven, earth, human beings and spirit have all got these two qis, Yin and Yang, which means that they have within them the exchange of qis.

Yin and Yang, which serve as links among sub-systems and factors and act among them, reach a relative balance and harmony of evolution through a long period of linking and acting. The balance of these two qis (Yin and Yang) within the body, is shown as the harmony and order of qi among the inner bodily organs and between the main and collateral energy-passing channels.

Subsequently, the physical body will achieve a peaceful and healthy state. The human body is an open system, constantly exchanging material, energy and messages with its surroundings. The changes in stars and the sun, the excessive or meagre amount on earth of the climatic 'six qis' (wind, cold, heat, humidity, dry and fire), and superiority or inferiority of food, air and water, and the stimulation received from social relationships will all influence (directly or indirectly in terms of qi) the mutual balance of Yin and Yang within the human body, and interfere with harmony and order of inner bodily organs and the main and collateral energy-passing channels.

Generally speaking, the potential power of the human physique will to some extent adapt the levels of Yin and Yang within the body to outside influences, to keep a relative balance, which is what we mean by keeping fit. But when that potential power becomes insufficient, or the outside interference gets too strong, bodily health is upset. The relative balance of Yin and Yang within the body is lost. The previous order of the inner bodily organs becomes disrupted and health turns into disease.

Tai-chi lays great emphasis upon Yin and Yang. As we have already discussed, by such activities as body adjustment, mind adjustment and breath adjustment, tai-chi actively strengthens that potential power in order to keep fit. This is what *Huang Di Nei Jing* refers to in the words, 'consolidation of spirit within drives away disease' and 'the positive qi within the body can keep disease away'. When the body's health has acquired great stability, the body will be able to deal with inside and outside interferences that would otherwise disturb the balance and order concerned with Yin and Yang.

These are some of the advantages tai-chi has over other sports. Its disease-curing function also lies in its balanced and harmonious movements, which are in agreement with the biological principles of the body and thus gradually adjust the unbalanced Yin and Yang (and the disorder of the organs' operations).

During the long process of evolution, mankind has acquired powers to resist disease, for example, through resistance to stimuli, immunity etc. Tai-chi, because it helps to increase the positive qi of the body, is a means to raise the individual's power against disease. Tai-chi's function – to build up health and cure disease – conforms with the Chinese traditional medical theory.

10 Fact, Fiction, Myth and Legend

Traditional taijiquan (the modern spelling of tai-chi-chuan), which may take 25 minutes to perform and contains many repeat movements. Cheng-man Ching formulated the 37-step (known as the short form) from the Yang style, and with students throughout the world it received much acclaim and is now widely practised.

The national sport of China is called wu-shu (martial art); in Taiwan they call it guo-shu (national art). The Chinese have stated that wu-shu will be included in the projected program for the Olympic games in the year 2000. The 1936 Olympics were the scene for the first world demonstration of these martial skills. Mr Zhang, the president of the Peking Physical Culture Institute, where I studied in 1981, was a member of the troupe who exhibited these ancient martial arts skills.

Nowadays in China, tai-chi is part of the program for wu-shu students on scholarships. They first learn the 24-step method (the one shown in this book) which takes about five minutes to perform, then they study the 48-step, which includes elements of the Chen style, then the short Chen form itself, and finally taijijien (tai-chi sword). Should their interest take them further, there is then a 66- and 88-step which are basically Yang style.

By the inclusion of the word 'chuan' or 'quan' which translates as 'fist' or 'boxing' method, taijiquan fully qualifies as a martial art, although in terms of acquiring the skill it is said to take about ten years before you can go out of the door 'with taijiquan', which means that it takes a long time before the martial skills are fully developed.

Apart from the solo exercise and pushing hands practice, there are three weapons in traditional taijiquan: the sword (jien), the cutlass (dao), and the staff (gan). The Chinese claim the sword is a scholar's weapon, likening the use of the sword to that of the calligrapher's brush. There are various areas along the blade which are functional in cutting. Many of the techniques are meant to attack your opponent's wrist and disarm him.

The dao or cutlass is another weapon which is practised within the tai-chi syllabus, but it seems to lack the popularity of the sword among practitioners. The big knife, as it is also termed, involves a movement which brings it over the head. This movement is not performed with the sword because it is a double-sided blade.

The third weapon is the staff, which involves a method of sparring practice involving the striking of staffs together in a circular motion.

The solo form, sword, cutlass and staff, along with the two-man exercise, make up this method of Chinese gung fu.

Tai-chi is practised widely in China from one end of the country to the other and has millions of followers. Japan now has close to a million adherents. Interestingly the Chen style with its more vigorous techniques and stamping seems to be gaining in popularity and perhaps is more suited to the national psyche.

There is a legend in tai-chi regarding an old master whose skill was so high that a bird could not alight on his hand because he was able to apply 'sticking energy' to the bird's feet and refuse to give purchase to the bird's attempt to alight. This may be put in the category of catching flies with chopsticks, but reflects the Chinese approach to skill being refined to its highest level.

One ancient master whose son led a life of debauchery locked him in a room for five years and daily visited him to teach him tai-chi pushing hands. One can only imagine his need to improve. Finally he was able to fight his way out past his father and he was reputed to be a reformed character.

Another ancient master was said to have chalked circles on the palms of his students' hands and during sparring sessions was able to witness their success by the marks left on each other's jackets.

There are many stories of tai-chi masters being able to uproot or lift or throw their opponents yards into the air, and tai-chi history abounds with stories of masters who were considered peerless in their time.

11 Qigong

Qigong (breath skill) is the collective name for a multitude of Chinese health skills which have been practised for over 3000 years. Paintings have been unearthed from the 4th century BC which show people performing various movements for health.

Qigong history can be divided into five historical branches: Buddhist, Taoist, Confucianist, martial arts and health. All deal with the movement of qi throughout the body using different methods and practices. Qigong skills were often the province of the shaman (witch doctor) and were guarded secrets, often used to control and enslave simple folk.

The Chinese martial arts have always proclaimed the benefits of qigong, not only to develop the 'iron-shirt' method whereby the practitioner is able to withstand the point of spears to the throat and crushing blows to the body, but also as a balance to the hard training that shaolin boxing demands.

In 1986 the Chinese sent a troupe of hard style qigong experts to demonstrate their skill before Western audiences. Bending iron bars, having bricks broken over their heads and striking themselves with swords did little to capture the imagination of an audience brought up to view such things as belonging to a circus and not as a science.

The 1949 revolution and the ensuing cultural revolution dispensed with the mystical appendages, and since 1980 qigong has been actively promoted by the government to the people.

It is reckoned that modern physiotherapy, which was created by the Swedish pioneer P. H. Ling, was stimulated by the Jesuit translations of Chinese philosophy. This knowledge of Chinese therapeutic gymnastics has become very important in the development of this remedial science.

Acupuncture, ginseng and qigong have long been considered panacea (cureralls) in Chinese culture. To give qigong its correct title would be to refer to it as kinesiatrics, which means the curing of illness through muscular movement.

Hospitals and research centres have sprung up in China since 1980 and many claims are being laid of various illnesses that have succumbed to the regular practice of this method. Patients are taught exercises that influence their particular illness. This holistic approach, in that the patient is part of the healing process, has met with wide acceptance. Some people have found that they can emit qi energy and there are a number of clinics that offer transmission therapy by a practitioner. Just as here in the West spiritual healing and radiance therapy have become popular of recent times, qigong in China has begun a renaissance of interest.

Medical qigong consists of meditation, postures and gentle movements. One recent method which is receiving great acclaim is the dayan gong (wild goose method) which is taught by Yang Meu Jeun, a 96-year-old woman who inherited the method from her grandfather. She spends much of her time diagnosing illnesses in hospitals, and it is claimed that when she transmits energy through her hands the scent of flowers may be smelled.

It would seem that the health-giving benefits of soft style qigong will receive a more welcome audience, as the population in the West is ageing, and people are becoming more suspicious of the pharmaceutical industry.

Tai-chi qigong is the bridge between these two ancient disciplines and allows people to practise a simpler method of exercise and so derive benefit much quicker, while taking some of the elements from tai-chi. Tai chi qigong contains 18 movements which are practised in a repeated manner, thereby encouraging the flow of qi through the body. This method was taught on Chinese television and received great acclaim.

Tai-chi qigong does not have any difficult steps and each movement involves the whole body. I would recommend that anyone undertaking a study of tai-chi first learn the tai-chi qigong, primarily because it is useful for the beginning student to learn the 18 movements individually and practise them first in front of a mirror. This initially builds confidence, and makes the learning of the more complicated 24-step much easier.

After practising tai-chi qigong sit down quietly and feel the glow of energy that you have created.

There is a method of acupuncture which treats the body through needling the ear. One of my teachers drew my attention to this and explained that if you rub your ears very gently for a few minutes when you are cold it will cause your whole body to become warm. I have found this also works, but there are longer lasting effects to be found in practising tai-chi qigong, along with improved health.

A friend of mine is a professional boxer who runs daily at 6 a.m. and has always suffered from cold hands. I showed him the tai-chi qigong and he practises them daily before his run. He now informs me that his hands remain warm throughout his morning training.

In winter many old people suffer from hypothermia. I'm sure that practising tai-chi qigong will help prevent this by circulating the qi and in doing so move the blood more freely to the extremities of the body.

I find it rewarding when an old person attends a class and after one session can feel improvement and a sense of accomplishment. This is due to the simplicity of the movements, whereas in the study of tai-chi it can take some time before the student (of any age) grasps the technique. This I feel has held back the development of tai-chi in the West, together with the lack of teachers. Even the Chinese attempts to simplify tai-chi by introducing the 24-step have not overcome the problem; the introduction of tai-chi qigong overcame this by allowing a direct interface with the movement.

Practising outside in clement weather is great fun and allows you to draw qi from the sky which is termed the 'great qi'. Learning a few movements and then practising them outside in the garden or in a secluded spot gives a functional reason to be there and allows you to receive 'earth qi' also. Imagine yourself as the antenna between the earth and sky and bring your body to a state of balance. If you practise regularly (whenever possible outside) you will feel stronger and will notice an improvement in your energy level. It is my dream that one day tai-chi qigong will be available in hospitals as treatment or part treatment for various conditions, and for groups to develop so that people of all ages may mix and practise together in a healthy atmosphere.

Added to each of the following exercises are the health benefits and the illness which benefits from the practise. Unlike tai-chi, tai-chi qigong begins each movement with the legs straight. Perform each of the movements in a smooth continuous action. To gain maximum benefit relax your fingers, wrists, elbows, shoulders and waist, do not overreach and slowly build up the movements to six or ten. Repeat each exercise, practise regularly and you will soon begin to feel the benefits of this treasure of Chinese health.

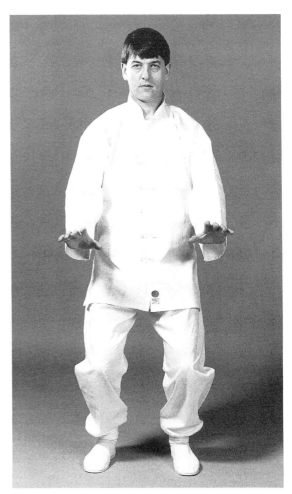

Fig. 1

STARTING POSITION

1: Movement description

Stand naturally with the legs shoulder width apart. Close the mouth. Drop and relax the shoulders. Keep the hips straight and the gravity in the centre. Slowly raise the arms to shoulder height. Then, whilst lowering the body and bending the knees, bring the arms down, exhaling on the downward movement and inhaling on the upward.

Repeat the exercise six times.

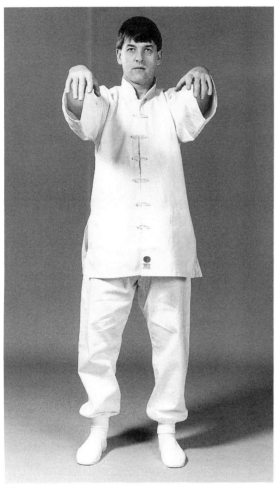

Fig. 2

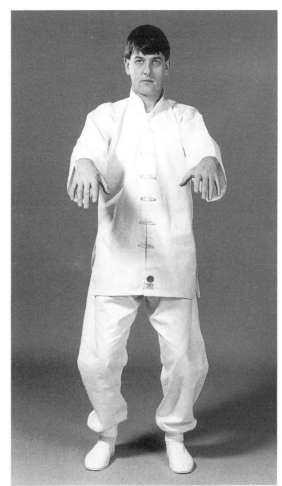

Fig. 3

2: Points to note

Before commencing the exercise it is advised to stand quietly in the standing posture for a few minutes in order to allow your body to relax. Keep the hips in a straight line with the body. Keep the head erect. Allow the elbows, wrists and fingers to bend naturally throughout the exercise. Let the arm movements follow the body in a coordinated manner.

3: Health benefits

This exercise is designed to balance the blood pressure and strengthen the heart. The gentle flexing movements of the shoulders, elbows, wrists, fingers and knees smooth the channels of energy and help prevent arthritis.

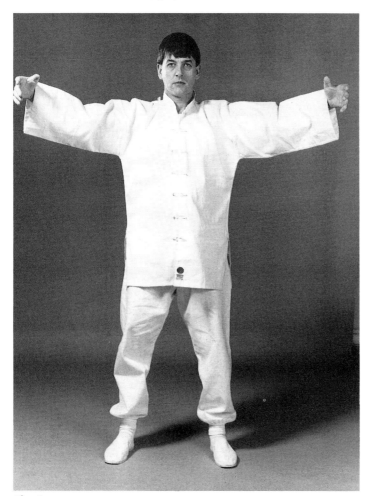

Fig. 1

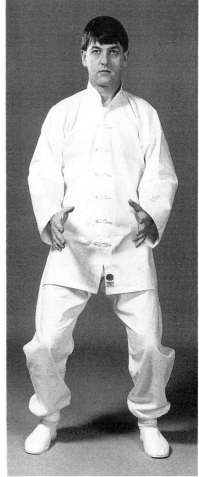

Fig. 2

OPENING THE CHEST

1: Movement description

Stand naturally, with your legs straight. Raise your hands to the front of your chest. Separate your arms to the side as you open your chest and breathe in. Bring the hands back to the body in a circling motion, finishing with the hands in front of the stomach, as you bend your legs and breathe out.

2: Points to note

When your hands are at chest height both body and legs straighten up at the same time. When the hands sink in front of your stomach your legs need to bend at the same time. Up and down, bend and straighten, breathe in, breathe out in coordination.

3: Health benefits

This exercise is beneficial for those suffering from depression, insomnia and hypertension.

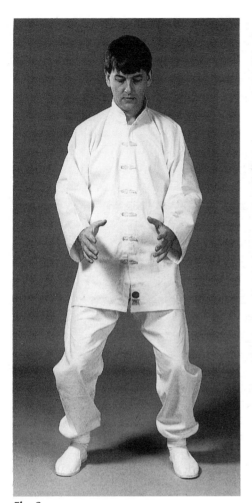

Fig. 3

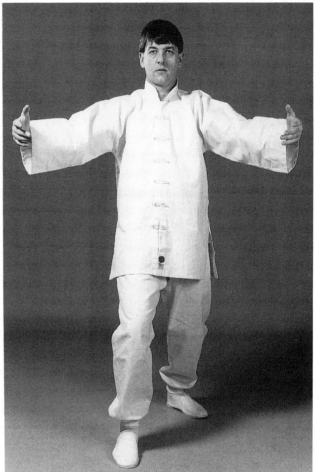

Fig. 4

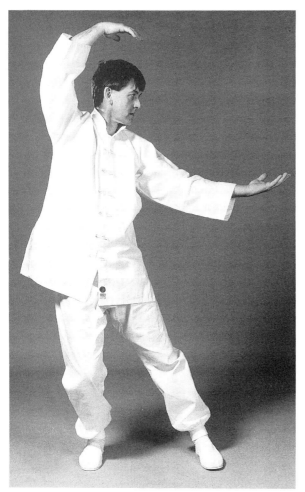

Fig. 1

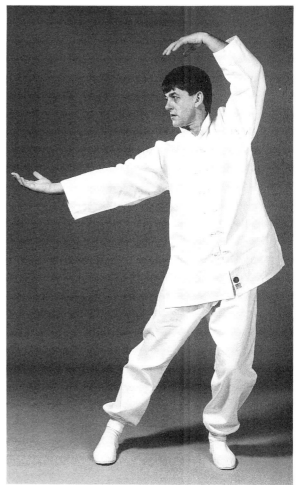

Fig. 2

RAINBOW DANCE

1: Movements description

a) Raise up both hands to the front of the chest, straighten the legs and bring both hands over the head, straightening the arms. Palms should face each other; breathe in.

b) Move your weight to the right leg, bending the knees at the same time. Straighten the left leg and raise the heel off the floor so that only the sole and toes are touching the floor. Bring the left hand down to the horizontal level of the left side, with the palm facing upward. The right arm arches a semi-circle bringing the right palm over the head. As the whole body moves to the right side, breathe in.

c) Repeat the above exercise on the opposite side, swaying gently from side to side in a smooth continuous motion.

Perform the exercise six times.

2: Points to note

The hand movements should be coordinated with the breathing, and the movement should have a gentle and flowing appearance.

3: Health benefits

This exercise is designed to balance the blood pressure, aid the digestive system and relieve stomach ache.

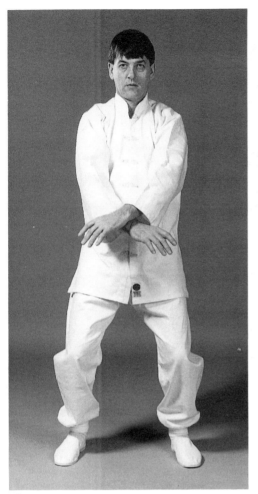

Fig. 1

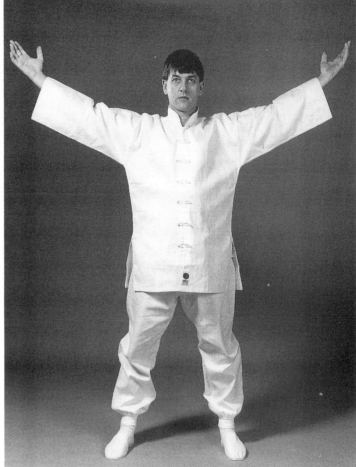

Fig. 2

SEPARATING CLOUDS BY WHEELING ARMS

1: Movement description

a) From a natural standing position bend both knees slightly. In doing so you are lowering the gravity and adopting a straddle/horse stance. At the same time place both hands in front of the body, palms facing the stomach. Raise both arms up over the head and separate, bringing them down and around back to the front of the stomach.

b) The legs bend as the arms come down, and straighten as the arms cross, and the palms circle outward and upward over the head.

2: Points to remember

Breathe in on the upward movement and out on the downward movement, remembering to keep the shoulders relaxed throughout. As the arms cross it is unimportant whether the hand is left over right or vice versa.

3: Health benefits

This exercise is useful in strengthening the legs, stimulating the kidneys and is beneficial for those suffering from neurasthenia.

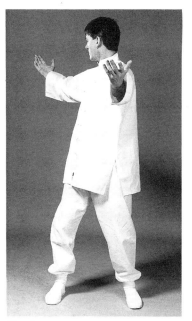
Fig. 1

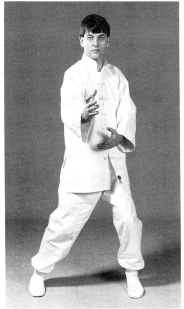
Fig. 2

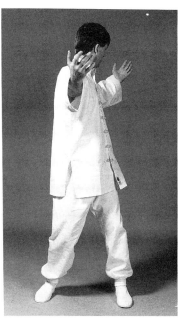
Fig. 3

ROLLING ARMS

1: Movement description

a) Begin by standing with the left hand extended palm upward in front of the body at chest height, the right hand raised to the side of the body, with the elbow bent and the hand at ear level. Push the right hand forward and down, simultaneously withdrawing the left hand so that the palms cross in front of the body. Turning the waist to the left causes the weight to transfer to the right leg, allowing the arms to freely extend.

b) Bring the left palm past the ear, down and through the centre, over the right palm, whilst withdrawing the right hand. Then transfer the weight to the other foot whilst turning the waist and extending the hands in the opposite direction. This completes the cycle to the opposite side.

2: Points to note

As the hands extend, inhale; as the hands ·cross and push forward, exhale. The centre of gravity should move between both legs and coordinate the waist with the movement of the legs. The movement should flow from one side to the other. If your posture, movement and breathing are correct you should experience a tingling sensation in your fingers.

3: Health benefits

This exercise benefits sufferers of neurasthenia, arthritis and asthma.

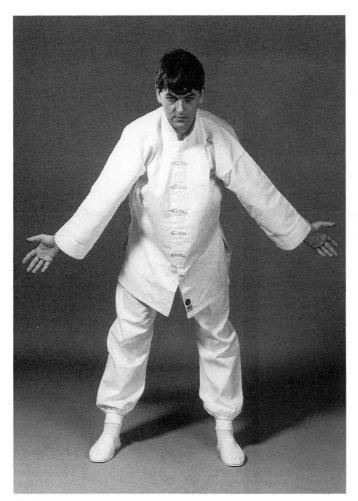

Fig. 1

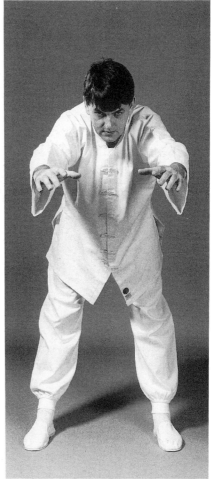

Fig. 2

ROWING THE BOAT IN THE CENTRE OF THE LAKE

1: Movement description

a) Stand naturally with your legs straight and bring your arms straight up from the side to the front and round over the top of the head. Gradually lean forward from the waist as your hands come around and down.

2: Points to note

As the hands come around and forward in front of the head keep the arms straight and the palms facing forward. As the arms are rolling keep them relaxed, as the waist bends forward breathe out. As the body straightens breathe in.

Practice this exercise six to ten times.

3: Health benefits

This exercise aids the digestive system, and is beneficial for those suffering from back-ache and headache.

155

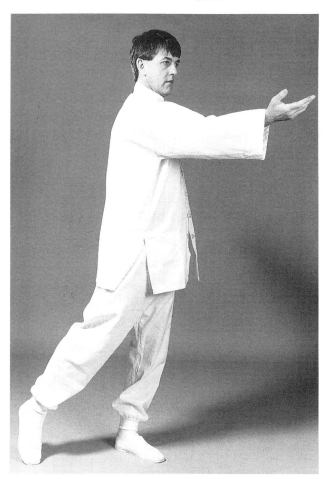

Fig. 1

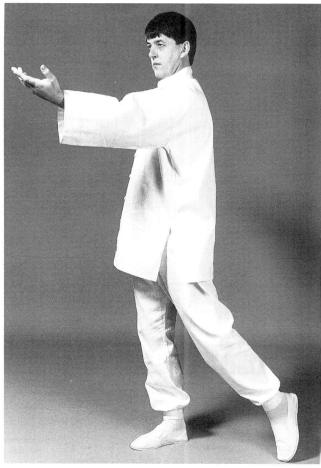

Fig. 2

LIFTING THE BALL IN FRONT OF THE SHOULDER

1: Movement description

a) Stand naturally, turn and lift the right palm upward to the left side of the body above shoulder height. Imagine you are lifting up a ball. Keep the left hand to the side of the body whilst moving your weight onto the left leg. The right leg stretches on to tiptoes with the heel up. Turn the waist and breathe in.

b) Changing from one side to the other, breathe in on the rising movement and out on the downward.

2: Points to note

When lifting up the ball, do it slowly. Imagine a real ball on your palm. Let the breathing naturally follow the movement. Practising this movement will allow you to feel the qi moving in your fingers.

3: Health benefits

By focusing the eyes on the upward hand it is possible to induce a state of self hypnosis. It is also beneficial for those suffering from insomnia and helps balance the blood pressure.

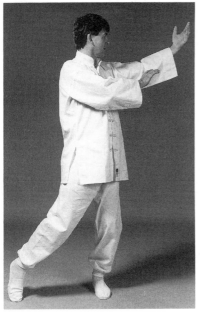

Fig. 1

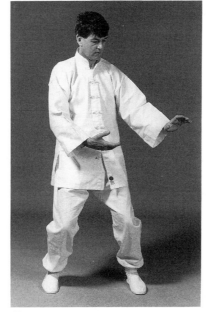

Fig. 2

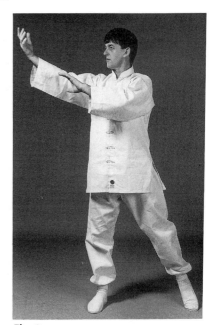

Fig. 3

LOOKING AT THE MOON BY TURNING THE BODY

1: Movement description

a) Adopt a standing position with your arms at your side. Keeping your arms straight, turn your body to the left and swing both arms along a parallel path upwards and to the side, allowing your right elbow to bend naturally, left palm facing up, right palm facing down.

b) Repeat this movement both sides, and practise the exercise eight to ten times.

2: Points to note

As you wave your arms upward look up and behind to the open palm. Transfer the weight smoothly from side to side. Bend the legs as the arms reach the downward position in the central changing posture.

3: Health benefits

This exercise stimulates blood circulation and slims the waist and hips. It is also beneficial for those suffering from neurasthenia.

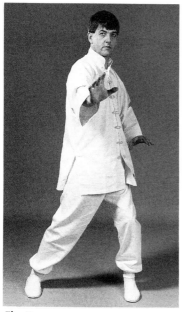

Fig. 1

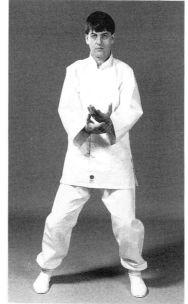

Fig. 2

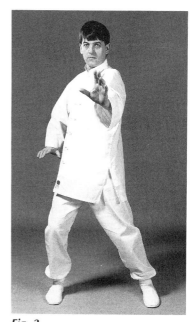

Fig. 3

PUSHING PALMS WHILST TURNING THE WAIST

1: Movement description

a) Stand naturally, adopt the horse-riding position and hold both hands palm upwards at the waist. Draw back the left hand slightly and turn the waist to the left. Turn and push forward with the right palm, bringing the left palm down to the side of the body and changing the balance to the left leg.

b) Turning, twisting and transfering the weight, bring the palms to cross over each other on the change-over from one side to the other. Keep the upper body steady as the waist turns to the side. Keep the tiger mouth open.

This exercise is repeated four times each side.

2: Points to note

Keeping the thumb and the forefinger stretched apart creates a tiger's mouth and opens and stimulates the 'valley' channel, which is located between the thumb and forefinger.

3: Health benefits

This exercise strengthens the spleen and also serves to promote leg and back energy.

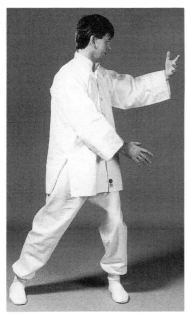
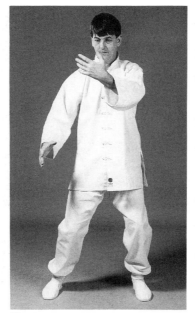
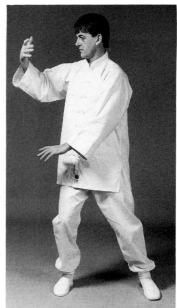

Fig. 1   Fig. 2   Fig. 3

CLOUD HANDS IN HORSE STANCE

1: Movement description

a) This exercise is the same as the Yang-style tai-chi waving hands in the clouds, except it is practised in a static position. Adopting the horse stance, turn the left palm inside up to face height, bringing the right hand across the front at waist height. Turn the waist to the left, and at the edge of the movement turn the left hand downward and bring the right hand facing upward.

b) Bring the waist around to the right; drawing the right palm across in front of the face, and scoop the left hand downward and across the body to the right side.

Repeat the exercise eight times.

2: Points to note

Let your breath naturally follow the movements as they interchange, forming two opposite turning and circling movements. Bring both arms to move in harmony with the eyes, following the upward hand. The weight moves from side to side in a fluid motion.

3: Health benefits

This exercise aids the digestive system and helps prevent arthritis.

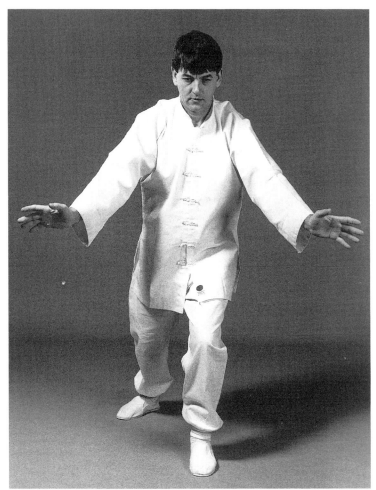

Fig. 1

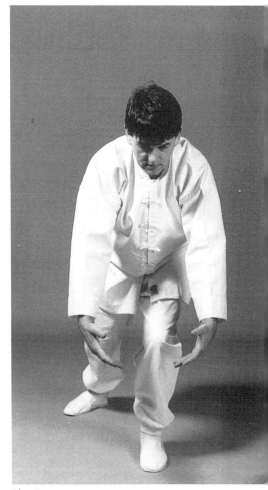

Fig. 2

SCOOPING THE SEA WHILE LOOKING AT THE SKY

1: Movement description

a) Put the left leg forward, making the bow step. Lean your body forward, bringing both hands to cross in front of the knee. Breathe out at the same time.

b) Crossing the hands they continue to follow the body as the gravity changes to the back leg. The hands open and separate, and the head finally looks at the sky as you breathe in. As the body changes to come forward, you breathe out and the hands gradually sink in front of your knee again.

Repeat the exercise with the opposite stance. Practise three to four times each way.

2: Points to note

As your body leans forward, your back leg straightens as your front leg bends. Bend your body forward as much as you comfortably can. When looking at the sky extend your arms outward with slow natural breathing.

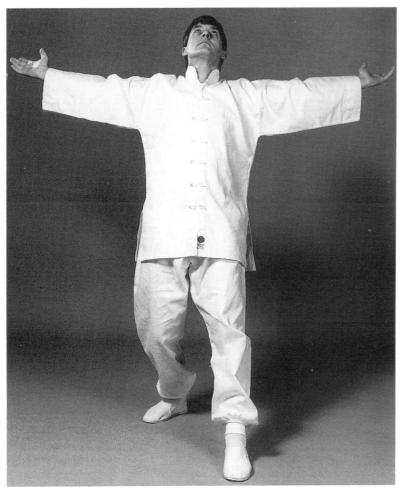

Fig. 3

3: Health benefits

Practising this exercise induces the muscles to relax, improves the blood circulation and balances the blood pressure.

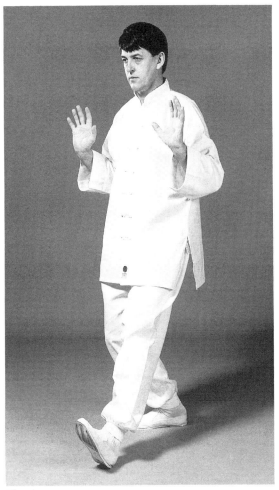

Fig. 1

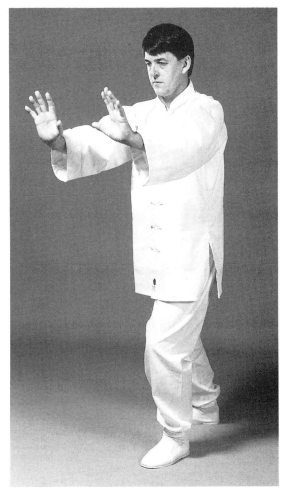

Fig. 2

PUSHING WAVE

1: Movement description

a) Stand in the bow stance with the right foot forward. Lift your palms up to the side of your chest, facing forward. Place the weight on the right foot and push forward with both palms at shoulder height. At the same time stretch the back leg, bringing it to a heel-raised position. Breathe out.

b) Slowly move your weight to the back leg and bring your forward foot to a toes-up position. Withdraw your arms while breathing in.

c) Change the leg position and practise three to four times each side.

2: Points to note

Remember to sink your elbows and shoulders and alternate the balance between the two legs smoothly. Use the mind, not force, to push the palms forward. When the palms retreat, imagine you are pressing down.

Beginners note: When moving back be careful not to overbend the back knee until your body is stronger.

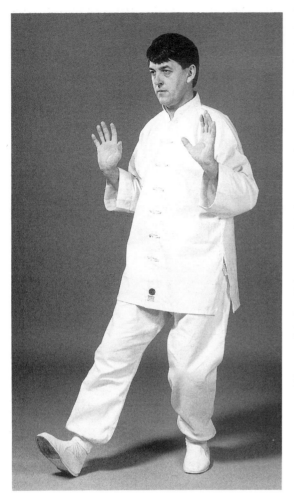

Fig. 3

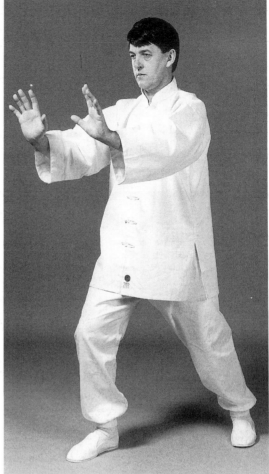

Fig. 4

3: Health benefits

This exercise strengthens the waist and leg energy and is beneficial for those suffering from hypertension.

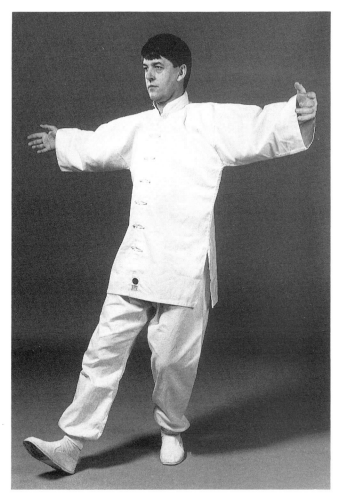

Fig. 1

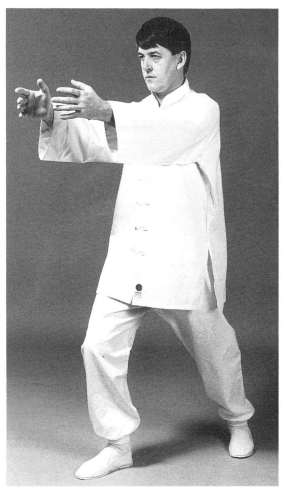

Fig. 2

FLYING PIGEON

1: *Movement description*

a) With one leg forward lift up both arms to the side. Place your weight on the back leg, lift up the toes of the front leg and breathe in, while you stretch out your hands imagine you are stretching something. Breathe in.

b) Transfering the weight to the front leg raise the heel of the back foot as you bring your hands together in front of the chest, breathe out.

c) Repeat the exercise three to four times each side.

2: *Points to note*

When the body leans back the arms are like the movements of a bird's wings. As the body moves forward both hands complete the movement with the palms facing. Remember to keep the arms, balance, breathing and movement coordinated.

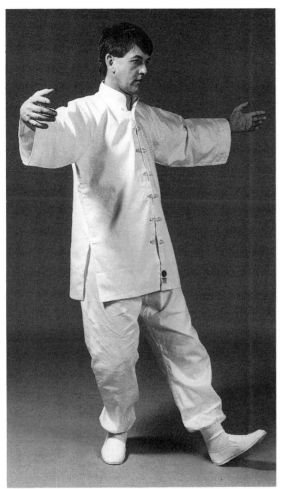

Fig. 3

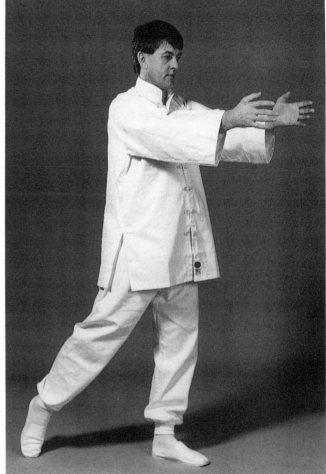

Fig. 4

3: Health benefits

This exercise is good for breathing, dispels feelings of oppression in the chest and promotes the digestive system.

165

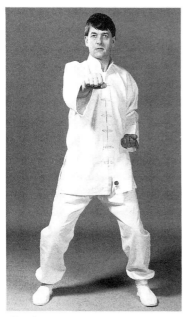
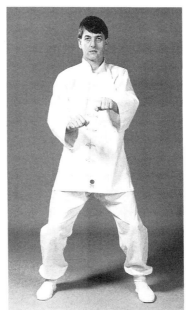
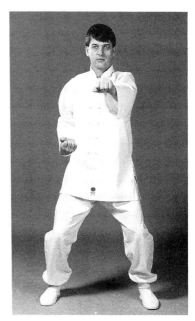

Fig. 1 *Fig. 2* *Fig. 3*

PUNCHING IN HORSE STANCE

1: Movement description

a) Adopt the straddle legged position, hold both fists under the armpit, then push out left hand, twisting the fist so that it finishes palm down. Withdraw the left hand as you push out the right. Keep the eyes focussed forward.

b) Practise the exercise ten times.

2: Points to note

Although this may resemble a martial method of punching, the breathing is different: in this method, there is inhalation at the end of the punch and breathing out at the change. Remember to keep your back straight, do not lean forward, and let the movements smoothly interchange.

3: Health benefits

This exercise promotes all round strength in the body and is invigorating practice.

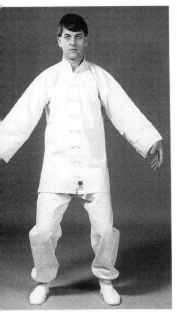

Fig. 1

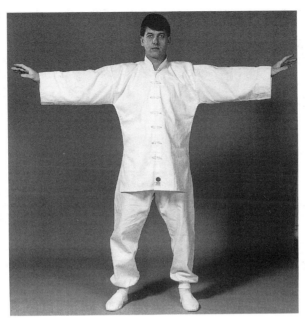

Fig. 2

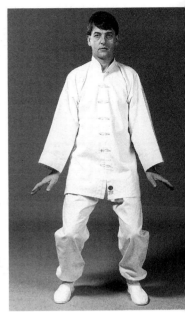

Fig. 3

FLYING WILD GOOSE

1: Movement description

a) Stand naturally, both hands raised up to shoulder height at the side of the body, then slowly squat down to horse stance. Let both hands drop down to the side like a big wild goose.

b) When you raise up the body, both hands raise to shoulder height. Breathe in on the upward movement and out on the downward movement.

Repeat the exercise eight times.

2: Points to note

You need to practise slowly so that your breathing does not become irregular. Move the arms in the action of a bird's wings and let the body movement lead the arms.

3: Health benefits

This exercise strengthens the kidneys and legs, improves low blood pressure and balances the blood pressure.

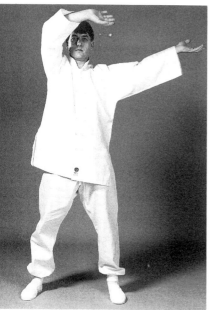
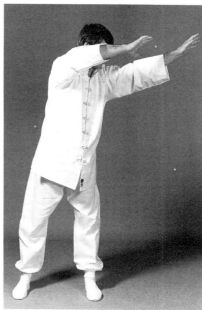
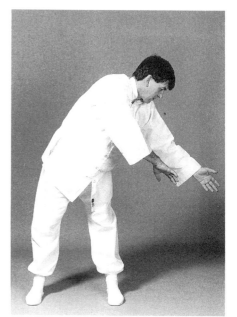

Fig. 1   Fig. 2   Fig. 3

ROTATING WHEEL IN A CIRCLE

1: Movement description

a) Stand naturally, bring both hands to cross in front of the stomach. Turn to the left side, keeping your arms straight. The arms follow the waist movement, moving upward around over the top of the head, palms facing forward. Breathe in at the same time. As the hand drops down the other side breathe out.

Repeat the exercise four to ten times each side.

b) Repeat in the opposite direction.

2: Points to note

While rotating the waist, the arms follow the movement and both palms face the same direction.

3: Health benefits

This exercise, practised slowly, is good for those suffering from low blood pressure. It also helps in the recovery of a tired body and reduces stiffness in the back.

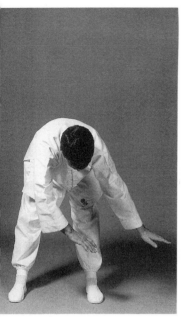

Fig. 4

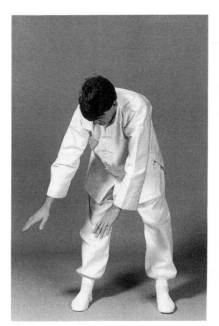

Fig. 5

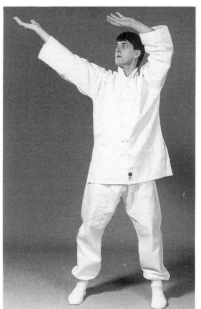

Fig. 6

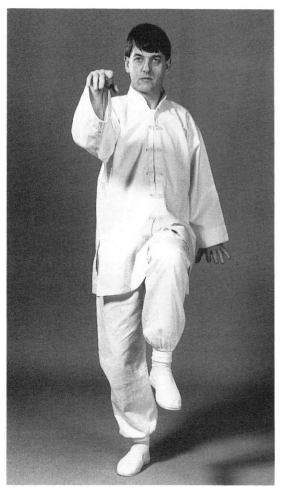

Fig. 1

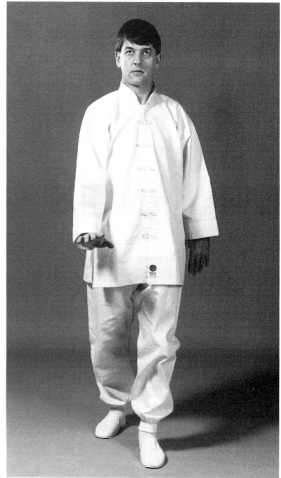

Fig. 2

MARCHING BOUNCING BALL

1: Movement description

a) From a natural position lift up the left leg. At the same time lift the right hand to shoulder height. Imagine bouncing a ball downward. Breathe in, and as you bring them down breathe out.

b) Repeat on opposite sides.

2: Points to note

Whilst performing this exercise – left hand, right leg, right hand, left leg – let the breathing naturally follow the movement.

Repeat the exercise eight to ten times.

3: Health benefits

This exercise is good for relaxing the body and recovering from tiredness.

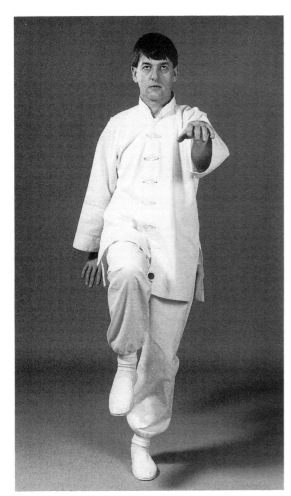

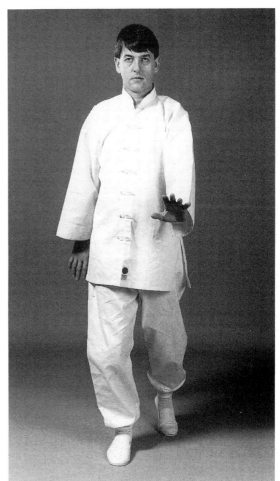

Fig. 3

Fig. 4

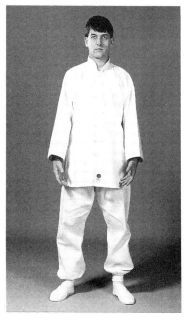

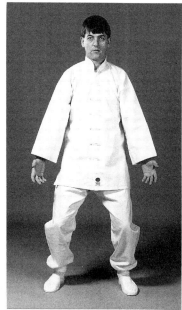

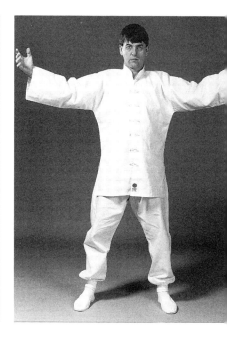

Fig. 1   Fig. 2   Fig. 3

SHAU GONG (BALANCING QI)

1: Movement description

a) Stand naturally, lift both hands palm upwards in front of the stomach, fingers to fingers. Lift the hands to the chest, breathe in and lift the heels.

b) Turn the palms down, keeping the fingers facing. Bring down the arms, from up to down to the dantien. Meanwhile breathe out and bring your heels down.

Repeat the exercise three to ten times.

2: Points to note

When the body is raised, breathe in; when down, breathe out.

No matter what movements you practise, you must finish with this exercise.

3: Health benefits

As the exercise is for calming down and balancing the qi, practice of this exercise alone gives great benefit.

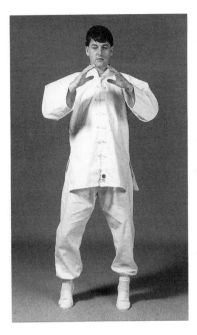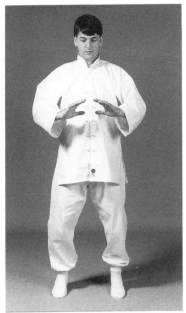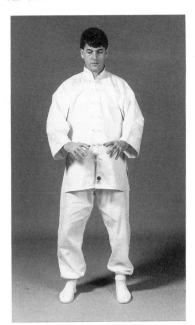

Fig. 4   Fig. 5   Fig. 6

These are the 18 tai-chi qigong. A full round of these exercises give a beneficial twenty minutes of stimulating exercise. You can practise in the home as little space is required. Doing the movements separately is OK and does no harm.

The best time to practise is in the morning in the fresh air. When you feel tired you can practise some of the movements to refresh your energy.

Each movement practised two to three times will take three to four minutes to complete. Regular practice will bring good health.

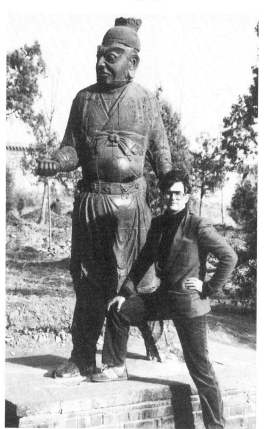

MARNIX WELLS

Marnix Wells was born in 1945, and attended Orwell Park School (near Ipswich) and Wellington College in Berkshire. In 1964 he went up to Oriel College, Oxford to read Oriental Studies. Between 1968 and 1971, Marnix continued his studies in Hong Kong, Taiwan and Japan, and while teaching English, studied Chinese music and tai-chi under various teachers. He studied pushing hands and set-sparring in addition to basic form under Gan Xiaoahon (Taipei) and Zhang Yizhong (Tokyo). He earned his black-belt in Northern Shaolin from Ti Myongsu (disciple of the Shandong master, Lu Shuitiau), and is still working towards an ever fuller synthesis of hard and soft!

Marnix presently manages a shipping firm in Seoul, South Korea. In 1982, he married a Chinese girl, Tsui-Ying. They have one daughter, Sarah.

Marnix Wells with Sing dynasty cast-iron guardian deities on Songshan, China's 'Central Peak', near Shaolin Temple, in March 1983

MICHAEL TSE

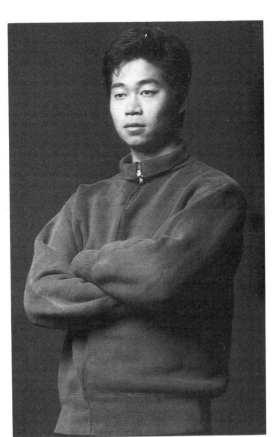

Michael Tse was born in Hong Kong and began studying the martial arts at the age of fifteen, under the guidance of his uncle, a herbalist and bonesetter. He is an 'indoor student' of Yip Chun (of the Wing Chun school), and also Yang Mei Jun, of the Dayan Gong school of Qigong.

He has studied and travelled extensively in mainland China, researching Feng Shui, I Ching and many aspects of Chinese culture. A former policeman in the Hong Kong Constabulary, Michael now conducts seminars and clinics in Europe and the United States. He is regarded by many as the foremost exponent of qigong in the western world.

Other Books on Tai-chi

Grateful thanks to Oriental World, Manchester, for supplying the following books:

1. Cheng Man-ch'ing, *T'ai Chi Ch'uan, a simplified method of calisthenics for health and self-defence* (North Atlantic Books, California).
2. Cheng Man-ch'ing and Smith, Robert, *T'ai Chi, the 'Supreme Ultimate' Exercise for Health, Sport and Self-defense* (Charles E. Tuttle, Vermont).
3. Cheng Man-ch'ing, *Master Cheng's Thirteen Chapters on T'ai Chi Ch'uan* (Sweet Ch'i Press, New York).
4. *Chen Style Taijiquan* (Hai Feng Publishing Co., Hong Kong).
5. Chen Wei-Ming, *T'ai Chi Ch'uan Ta Wen, Questions and Answers on T'ai Chi Ch'uan* (North Atlantic Books, California).
6. Chia Siew Pong and Goh Ewe Hock, *T'ai Chi, Ten Minutes to Health* (Times Books International, Singapore).
7. Da Liu, *T'ai Chi Ch'uan and the I Ching* (Routledge and Kegan Paul, London).
8. Galante, Lawrence, *Tai Chi, the Supreme Ultimate* (Samuel Weiser, Maine).
9. Horwitz, Tem and Kimmelman, Susan, with H. H. Lui, *Tai Chi Ch'uan, the Technique of Power* (Rider & Co., London).
10. Huang, Al Chung-liang, *Embrace Tiger, Return to Mountain* (Real People Press, Utah).
11. Jou, Tsung Hwa, *The Tao of Tai Chi Chuan* (Charles E. Tuttle, Vermont).
12. Klein, Bob, *Movements of Magic, the Spirit of T'ai Chi Ch'uan* (Newcastle Publishing Co. Inc., California).
13. Laing, T. T., *T'ai Chi Ch'uan for Health, Self-Defense, Philosophy and Practice* (Vintage Books, New York).
14. Lee, Douglas, *T'ai Chi Chuan, the Philosophy of Yin and Yang and its Application* (Ohara Publications Inc., California).
15. Lo/Inn/Amacker/Foe, *The Essence of T'ai Chi Ch'uan* (North Atlantic Books, California).
16. Maisel, Edward, *Tai Chi for Health* (Holt, Rinehart and Winston).
17. *Simplified Taijiquan* (Hong Kong Publishing Co., Hong Kong).
18. Wen-Shan Huang, *Fundamentals of Tai Chi Ch'uan* (South Sky Book Co., Seattle and Hong Kong).
19. Wile, Douglas, *T'ai Chi Touchstones, Yang Family Secret Transmissions* (Sweet Ch'i Press, New York).
20. Yang Ming-Shi, *Illustrated Tai'Chi Chuan for Health and Beauty* (Bunka Publishing Co., Tokyo).
21. Howard Reid, *The Way of Harmony* (Unwin Hyman, London).